Viral Replication and Production

Edited by Imran Shahid
and Abdullah Rzgallah Alzahrani

Published in London, United Kingdom

Viral Replication and Production
http://dx.doi.org/10.5772/intechopen.1006251
Edited by Imran Shahid and Abdullah Rzgallah Alzahrani

Contributors
Abdullah R. Alzahrani, Ammara Chaudhry, Anil Gattani, Ashok Kumar, Danial Zareh, Danyue Qu, Davgadorj Chantsalmaa, Dheeraj Kumar, Giti Paimard, Hao Kang, Imran Shahid, Iqra Mushtaq, Junling Zhang, Muhammad Sajjad Sarwar, Priya Hays, Ram Kumar, Reyhaneh Nekounam Ghadirli, Saijun Fan, Sanju Mandal, Sen Wang, Sisi Chen, Tahereh Alinejad, Wenyan Wu, Xin Yan, Xinyuan Ji, Yang Liu, Yan Yan, Yingyi Zhang, Yunrui Ru, Yu Zhao, Zuo Hao

First published in London, United Kingdom, 2025 by IntechOpen
IntechOpen is the global imprint of INTECHOPEN LIMITED, registered in England and Wales, registration number: 11086078, 167-169 Great Portland Street, London, W1W 5PF, United Kingdom

For EU product safety concerns: IN TECH d.o.o., Prolaz Marije Krucifikse Kozulić 3, 51000 Rijeka, Croatia, info@intechopen.com or visit our website at intechopen.com.

British Library Cataloguing-in-Publication Data
A catalogue record for this book is available from the British Library

Viral Replication and Production
Edited by Imran Shahid and Abdullah Rzgallah Alzahrani
p. cm.
Print ISBN 978-1-83634-482-7
Online ISBN 978-1-83634-481-0
eBook (PDF) ISBN 978-1-83634-483-4

If disposing of this product, please recycle the paper responsibly.

Meet the editors

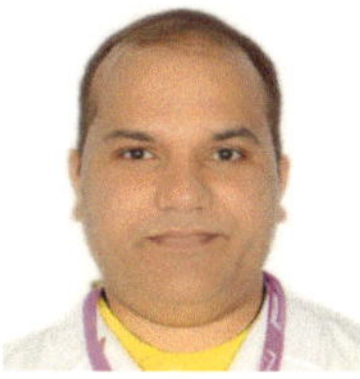

Imran Shahid, Ph.D., is an Associate Professor in the Department of Pharmacology and Toxicology, Faculty of Medicine, at the Umm Al-Qura University (UQU), Makkah, Saudi Arabia. He is a passionate academic, teaching various course modules in Health and Life Sciences to students in the Bachelor of Medicine & Bachelor of Surgery (MBBS) and Doctor of Pharmacy (PharmD) degree programs since 2012. He is also a prolific researcher in Molecular Biology, Molecular Virology, Molecular Pharmacology, and Cancer Therapeutics. His research focus lies in mapping host-virus networks in viral disease progression and the molecular basis of infectious viral diseases. He has published numerous research/review articles, as well as book chapters, and authored/edited two books on HCV-host interactions, HCV diagnosis, and its treatment.

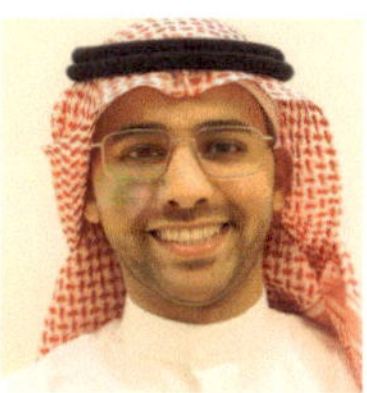

Dr. Abdullah R. Alzahrani is currently an associate professor and chairman of the Department of Pharmacology and Toxicology, Faculty of Medicine, at the Umm Al-Qura University (UQU), Makkah, Saudi Arabia. He completed his Ph.D. degree in Pharmacology and Toxicology from the University of Strathclyde, UK, in 2019. He is a productive researcher in pharmacology, with research interests focused on the development of novel drug delivery systems for breast cancer, colon cancer, and Alzheimer's disease. He is a member of the Saudi Toxicology Society, the Royal Pharmaceutical Society, the British Toxicology Society, and the Glasgow Pharmacological Society, among others. He is the author of many peer-reviewed research and review articles in prestigious and well-renowned international research journals.

Contents

Preface

The mechanisms and processes of viral replication and production remain mysterious, complex, and involve intricate interplays between host-virus genome/proteome interactions. Both phenomena also vary at the host cellular and molecular levels, based on virus classification/families, diverse viral genome configurations, and the players involved (e.g., virus- and host-specific proteins, a plethora of genes, and signaling cascades) when a virus replicates and produces new progeny. The quest to unfold and elucidate the unique viral replication strategies and novel viral progeny processes has fascinated virologists for decades. Similarly, the outcomes of these phenomena in a virus's life cycle are also vital for determining viral pathogenesis, viral infection kinetics/dynamics, and for developing effective antiviral treatments and preventive strategies. Similarly, the cusp of an Artificial Intelligence (AI), Deep Learning (DL), and Machine Learning (ML) revolution in the recent decade has also revolutionized viral genome-human proteome interactions by evolving huge datasets of viral replication and transcription processes to predict host cell infectivity, infection progression, emergence of viral variants, and prepardiness and management of possible viral outbreaks as future epidemics and pandemics.

Viral Replication and Production is divided into four sections. The first section is the introduction, which briefly explains the viral replication and production phenomena of certain human infectious disease-causing viruses. It also provides an overview of the foundational discussions in the remaining sections, and subsequent book chapters delve into various novel aspects of specific viruses. The second section unveils the unique viral replication mechanisms/strategies and adaptation techniques. This section also briefly represents viral immunopathogenesis and its pathogenic relevance. The third section elucidates the regulation of viral replication and production, and also provides insights into the biogenesis of infectious viral particles. The last (fourth) section of the book addresses novel approaches in the pipeline for therapeutic interventions of next-generation viral infections, as well as the latest advancements in artificial intelligence models/tools to predict viral genome-human proteome interactions and forecast future viral outbreaks. Beyond viral replication and production, this book also explores broader themes, including growth factors and radiation that regulate viral replication, as well as virion dynamics and genetic strategies for producing infectious viral particles.

This informative book is intended for a wide range of audiences, including viral pathologists, professionals, researchers, students, and virologists in the field. We are confident that the unique contents of this book, including an amalgamation of the latest advancements in biotechnology to study viral genome and human proteome interactions, will be valuable in conjunction with the innovative artificial intelligence predictive models to combat the emerging threats of viral pathogens in public health and to design preventive strategies for future viral epidemics and pandemics. We are incredibly grateful and pay our sincere gratitude to all the contributors from different parts of the world who are excellent researchers, renowned professionals, and instrumental thinkers in the field of virology. We hope that their dedication, novel ideas, and excellent scientific findings present a broader spectrum of their research vision and scientific knowledge about this hot spot issue in virology, sparking intellectual curiosity and understanding among newcomers in the field.

A long journey may be easier when traveling together, and interdependence often yields more valuable outcomes than independence does. During the development of this book, we were accompanied and supported by our colleagues at the Department of Pharmacology and Toxicology, Faculty of Medicine, Umm Al-Qura University, Makkah, Saudi Arabia. We take great pleasure in this moment to express our heartfelt gratitude to all of them for bringing this publication to fruition.

Finally, we dedicate this book to all those who have been affected by any type of virus, who are fighting against any viral infection, and to all the clinicians, health-care providers, physicians, paramedics, and medical residents who are always at the forefront to treat, manage, and prevent any viral outbreak as a potential endemic, epdiemic, or pandemic worldwide.

Imran Shahid, PhD and Abdullah R. Alzahrani, PhD
Faculty of Medicine,
Department of Pharmacology and Toxicology,
Umm Al-Qura University,
Makkah, Saudi Arabia

Section 1

Introduction

Chapter 1

Introductory Chapter: Viral Replication and Production Are Always Phenomenal for Viral Infections

Abdullah R. Alzahrani and Imran Shahid

1. Introduction

1.1 Viral replication mechanisms and virion formation processes are still mysterious and elusive

For the last two decades, the world has been under the siege of different viral epidemics and pandemics, which have disrupted the health of millions of humans and caused countless mortalities. Coronaviruses (CoVs), dengue virus (DENV), hepatitis C virus (HCV), Middle East respiratory syndrome (MERS) virus, and Zika virus are some examples of human disease-causing viruses that drastically shook the world and jolted even the best healthcare systems in developed and resource-rich nations in recent years. Albeit these viruses comprise different morphologies and classify into different families according to their taxonomical position, surprisingly, they share similar molecular biology in their hosts and, to some extent, viral infectivity mechanisms. Being an obligate parasite, a virus's life cycle in a host cell is either lysogenic or lytic and usually involves steps like attachment, penetration, uncoating, genome replication, transcription, translation, assembly, and release of the offspring virions [1]. Among these key steps of a virus life cycle, viral replication and biogenesis of the virion are prerequisites to generate highly mutated virus genomes, viral variants, and highly infectious viral particles to affect the adjacent host cells and transmit from one host to another. Subsequently, the viruses exhibit different replication mechanisms and use host cell machinery to accomplish these life cycle events and evolve diversity in their genetic makeup and adopt the capacities to translocate those variations to the next hosts (i.e., viral replication fitness) [2].

We have two broad classifications of viruses as RNA and DNA viruses, based on their genome composition; hence, each class is replicated by different replication enzymes. Similarly, the fidelity of replication enzymes also impacts the viral replication accuracy, efficiency, and maintains the genetic integrity of the parent viral genome [3]. These dynamics of the viral replication enzymes may favor rapid evolution of the viruses and the emergence of drug-resistant viral variants. However, the viral replication enzymes' kinetics/dynamics within the host cells' cytoplasm and nucleus, viral replication enzyme fidelities, and membraneous web formation for replication by certain viruses are still mysterious, murky, and yet to be fully elucidated both at the cellular and molecular levels. Similarly, the biogenesis of virion, the perplexing virion host immune evasion strategies, and the virion transmission to uninfected host cells also represent some key issues in the field of virology and eagerly demand to obtain the relevant answers with mechanistically thoughtful explanations.

The viral replication mechanisms are not so simple, and viral replication regulation by the host cellular proteins, cell signaling networks, and a plethora of genes is also a hot spot research topic. How the state-of-the-art microscopic techniques visualize the virion morphology, and how the advancements in radiation technologies have made it possible to explain the synergistic effects of oncolytic viruses to treat certain types of oncogenic-induced human cancers, also need further elucidation. Similarly, how the gene-level therapeutic approaches offer a new avenue for the control or treatment of certain infectious human viral infections (e.g., DENV) also needs to be fully investigated. Extensive studies are also needed to potentiate the role of computational virology, novel Artificial Intelligence (AI) tools, and improved Machine Learning (ML) models in the studies of viral genome-human proteome interactions, viral replication, transcription processes, and their ultimate impacts on viral infectivity.

2. Viral replication mechanisms and strategies are quite sophisticated and diverse

Virus replication relies on different factors, including genome composition, virus classification, and their dynamic interactions with the target hosts. RNA viruses replicate their genome in the host cytoplasm by an RNA polymerase enzyme, while most DNA viruses use DNA polymerases of their infected hosts to replicate in the host cell nucleus [4]. On the other hand, retroviruses, by using the phenomenon of reverse transcription, incorporate their viral genome into the genetic material of their hosts [5]. Although the viruses entirely depend on the host cells for replication, they exhibit notable diversity in how they do so.

Indeed, viral genomes are more diverse and highly variable than the genomes of cellular organisms, which generally comprise double-stranded DNA (dsDNA). However, viral replication strategies by and large depend on the type of host cell infected by a virus (either a eukaryotic or a prokaryotic host cell) [6]. It means that viruses adapt themselves to the varying cellular conditions within a host cell before initiating viral replication and formation of new virions. To regain this adaptability within a host cell, viruses have evolved a lot of tricks by using special replication enzymes, co-opting host translation and replication processes, and taking control of host cell machinery [7]. On the flip side of the coin, all viruses, either RNA or DNA, meet similar challenges during the formation of new virus particles, including the fidelity of their replication enzymes, accurate writing of their genome to synthesize essential viral proteins, and infallible post-translational modifications to assemble virions [8]. Importantly, viral infectivity, which is the outcome of a virus's life cycle within the host, primarily depends on viral replication rate, biogenesis of virion, and virion transmission to new hosts. Subsequently, the viral genome host proteome interactions, viral genome host immune evasion strategies, and rapid viral replication rate have devised an ongoing evolutionary arms race where the viruses evolve exceptional means to evade host immune control and emerge as the novel viral variants of concern (VOC; e.g., SARS-CoV-2) [9].

3. Both viral and host factors are essential for viral replication regulation

Virus-host dependencies are essential for virus replication and the production of new viral progeny, which ultimately infect other host cells and maintain viral infectivity [10]. Regardless of the viral determinants, the host cellular factors, cell signaling networks, and a plethora of host genes play an integral role in viral replication, virion formation, and transmission from an infected host to a healthy cell, tissue, or host (i.e., viral tropism) [11]. Viral tropism could be at the cellular, tissue, or host level and is determined by a combination of factors, including the availability of cellular proteins/receptors to which a virus can bind, compatibility of the intracellular environment for viral replication, and the virus's capability to evade the host's immune system responses. Furthermore, the propagation of an acute viral infection to the chronic stage and subsequently to the end-stage illnesses also relies on various host factors and key players to exacerbate viral proteins to take control of host cell machinery to disrupt normal cellular functions/processes [11].

Host cellular factors (e.g., proteins, receptors, growth factors) generally involved in regular functions of the cell crosstalk with virus proteins to support the viral replication and formation of new virus particles inside the host cells [10, 11]. Similarly, certain host DNA transcription and replication proteins modulation, cytokine gene polymorphism, alteration of host cell metabolome, and intracellular signaling also play a vital role in damaging the infected host cells by activating cell proliferation, prohibiting apoptosis of infected cells, and up- or down-regulation of host genes or protein functions to develop cell carcinogenesis [11].

4. Novel antiviral approaches and advancements in AI tools are vital to control future viral epidemics and pandemics

Viral infections are prevailing worldwide at higher rates despite the advent and approval of highly efficacious, well-tolerated oral antivirals, the accessibility of prophylactic and protective vaccines, and the availability of state-of-the-art diagnostic tools. Similarly, the evolution of lethal viral variants and the viral outbreaks in certain parts of the world also threaten to emerge as fatal viral epidemics or pandemics globally. Viral tropism, population demographics, infection epidemiology, inequity in diagnostic and treatment access, harder-to-reach vulnerable subpopulations, and socio-economic factors have played an integral role in spreading certain viral epidemics and pandemics over the last two decades in the world. Those viral outbreaks put high pressure on the best healthcare infrastructure in resource-rich nations and severely jolted the economies of developing and middle-income nations.

A key lesson learned while fighting against the COVID-19 pandemic in recent years was to tackle SARS-CoV-2 with multi-pronged strategies to inhibit viral replication and reduce transmission. During that period, the world has seen a rapid pace of advancements in viral genome sequencing techniques (i.e. spatial sequencing), the development of high-tech viral screening and diagnostic kits, emerging vaccine technologies, the design of state-of-the-art computational models for spatial viral analyses, and innovations in AI tools, ML models to oversee SARS-CoV-2 surveillance, COVID-19 spread, design healthcare strategies to treat and manage infection, and to forecast future pandemic events. Despite a significant role played by universal SARS-CoV-2 screening and vaccine campaigns to curb the pandemic, the extensive use of novel AI and ML models helped a lot to predict the viral genome-human proteome interactions, viral replication, and transcription processes, identification of novel drug targets, vaccine design models, viral infectivity analysis, and to define COVID-19 treatment and management guidelines/protocols.

A lot has been done in the screening, diagnosis, treatment, and management of various viral infections, including Dengue, HCV, HIV, MERS, SARS-CoV-2, and Zika in recent years while developing smart screening and diagnostic tools, the development of effective protective vaccines, and computational advancement in modulating the risk prediction tools and the mathematical modeling for a viral epidemic or pandemic preparedness. A lot will have to be done while developing novel gene-level antiviral therapeutics against viral infections, as well as inventing accurate, precise, and rich structural datasets, for AI, ML, and computational algorithms to forecast future viral epidemics and pandemics.

5. Conclusions

Viral replication mechanisms and production strategies teach valuable lessons about their survival, virulence, and further evolution as new viral variants. However, viruses are very smart at doing this and are masters of molecular adaptations. Viral replication fitness, the fidelity of virus polymerase enzymes, and viral mechanisms of host immune system evasion play a crucial role in those processes to happen. An ample understanding of the exact molecular connections of virus-host interactions and viral replication mechanisms, viral replication regulation, and immune system evasion strategies will open new avenues in the field of viral drug discovery to design more effective vaccines and antiviral therapies. Harnessing the unique capabilities of oncolytic viruses to selectively infect and destroy cancer cells, with the established efficacy of radiation, may offer a multifaceted approach to combat oncogenic virus-induced cancers. *Wolbachia*-based interventions offer a novel gene-level strategy to control next-generation dengue virus infection by reducing viral replication and disrupting the primary vector spread. The latest advancement in the development of AI tools, ML modeling, Computational Biology, and their subsequent use in virology research has generated a huge volume of data to illuminate virus-genome-human proteome interactions involving virus replication and transcription processes to predict viral infectivity and forecast the emergence of future viral outbreaks and reemergence of viral epidemics and pandemics.

Author details

Abdullah R. Alzahrani and Imran Shahid*
Department of Pharmacology and Toxicology, Faculty of Medicine, Umm Al-Qura University, Al-Abidiyah, Makkah, Saudi Arabia

*Address all correspondence to: iyshahid@uqu.edu.sa

References

[1] Koonin EV, Dolja VV, Krupovic M, Varsani A, Wolf YI, Yutin N, et al. Global organization and proposed megataxonomy of the virus world. Microbiology and Molecular Biology Reviews: MMBR. 2020;**84**(2):e00061-e00019. DOI: 10.1128/MMBR.00061-19

[2] Fornés J, Tomás Lázaro J, Alarcón T, Elena SF, Sardanyés J. Viral replication modes in single-peak fitness landscapes: A dynamical systems analysis. Journal of Theoretical Biology. 2019;**460**:170-183. DOI: 10.1016/j.jtbi.2018.10.007

[3] Xie Y, Kuai L, Peng Q, Wang Q, Wang H, Li X, et al. Structural basis of DNA replication fidelity of the Mpox virus. Proceedings of the National Academy of Sciences of the United States of America. 2025;**122**(10):e2411686122. DOI: 10.1073/pnas.2411686122

[4] Grellet E, L'Hôte I, Goulet A, Imbert I. Replication of the coronavirus genome: A paradox among positive-strand RNA viruses. The Journal of Biological Chemistry. 2022;**298**(5):101923. DOI: 10.1016/j.jbc.2022.101923

[5] Crater JM, Nixon DF, Furler O'Brien RL. HIV-1 replication and latency are balanced by mTOR-driven cell metabolism. Frontiers in Cellular and Infection Microbiology. 2022;**12**:1068436. DOI: 10.3389/fcimb.2022.1068436

[6] Aylward FO, Moniruzzaman M. Viral complexity. Biomolecules. 2022;**12**(8):1061. DOI: 10.3390/biom12081061

[7] Priyadarshi H, Das R. Complexities in viral replication strategies as a potential explanation for prevalence of asymptomatic carriers in Covid-19 infections: Analytical observation on SARS-Cov2 genome characteristics. Theory in Biosciences = Theorie in den Biowissenschaften. 2021;**140**(3):241-247. DOI: 10.1007/s12064-021-00349-3

[8] Cheng N, Liu M, Li W, Sun B, Liu D, Wang G, et al. Protein post-translational modification in SARS-CoV-2 and host interaction. Frontiers in Immunology. 2023;**13**:1068449. DOI: 10.3389/fimmu.2022.1068449

[9] Zupin L, Fontana F, Clemente L, Boschian-Bailo P, Ruscio M, Crovella S. Persistent viral infectivity after 27 days from COVID-19 symptoms onset. Journal of Clinical Pathology. 2022;**75**(3):211-214. DOI: 10.1136/jclinpath-2021-207394

[10] Speranza E. Understanding virus-host interactions in tissues. Nature Microbiology. 2023;**8**(8):1397-1407. DOI: 10.1038/s41564-023-01434-7

[11] AbuBakar U, Amrani L, Kamarulzaman FA, Karsani SA, Hassandarvish P, Khairat JE. Avian influenza virus tropism in humans. Viruses. 2023;**15**(4):833. DOI: 10.3390/v15040833

Section 2

Viral Replication and Production Mechanisms and Strategies

Chapter 2

Diversity of Viral Replication Strategies

Dheeraj Kumar

Abstract

Viruses are wonderful parasites that replicate and propagate within their host systems. Due to their host relationship, structural properties, and genomic structure decision, they can replicate in different organisms. The virus replication cycle involves steps like attachment, penetration, uncoating, genome replication, transcription, translation, assembly, and release of offspring virions. The viral families exhibit different methods to overcome these replication stages and show diversity and capacity to adapt to variations in their genetic makeup. RNA viruses often rely on enzymes made by viruses to copy RNA in the cytoplasm. On the other hand, DNA viruses use the DNA polymerases of the host (desired) in the nucleus. Retroviruses use reverse transcription to incorporate their genome into the DNA of their hosts. This book chapter gives a full survey of the diversity of viral replication strategies. It will highlight the differences between viral families and their dynamic interaction with their hosts. A complete understanding of viral replication strategies will help design and develop novel diagnostic tools, as well as antivirals and candidate vaccines.

Keywords: viral replication, genome diversity, DNA viruses, RNA viruses, replication strategies

1. Introduction

Ever since the tobacco mosaic virus (TMV) was discovered in 1892, the field of work in replication of virus technique has changed drastically. Scientists first studied bacteriophages because they helped study the cycles of viral reproduction. The electron microscopy invention (1930s) changed everything about viral architectures. Also, genome replication and expression of viruses were explained by the second half of the twentieth century with the help of molecular biology tools. Even though they appear to be simple parasites, viruses are among the most diverse and adaptable living things. Through millions of years, they have survived and evolved due to their ability to hijack the host's cellular machinery to replicate. Even though viruses are simple, they possess very sophisticated mechanisms to spread within their hosts. Viruses can adapt to almost any environment and can avoid the defense of almost all hosts [1]. Every virus's survival strategy involves repayment, and how it gets replicated varies from virus to virus. The kind of genome – DNA, RNA, or reverse-transcribing RNA – informs the replication processes and the degree to which host or viral enzymes are relied upon. The activities different viruses undergo and how they become infectious can affect whether the viruses will become pathogenic or not. Viruses are the most extreme of parasites. They have lost much of their genetic material to utilize the cellular machinery of their host. Yeast, which belongs to the fungus kingdom, is employed for fermentation in various industries, including sugar, milk, bacterial, and cytological [1]. Whatever their differences, all viruses require certain things to replicate successfully. Viruses are distinct life forms that do not fit within the definition of living things. Although viruses entirely rely on host cells for replication, they show notable diversity in how they do so. Viral genomes are highly variable, unlike the genomes of cellular species, which are generally all double-stranded DNA (dsDNA) [2].

Their life cycle can be linear or circular, single-stranded or double-stranded, composed of DNA or RNA, or both. Because of this variation in viral genome structure, viral replication is a very special and varied process. Since viral genomes have a lot of diversity, the viruses have to follow various host cell replication strategies that appropriately utilize cellular machinery. DNA viruses could depend more on their hosts' machinery, whereas RNA viruses may carry RNA-dependent RNA polymerase (RdRps) for assistance with genome copying. Viruses such as retroviruses also undergo reverse transcription, where their RNA genome is converted into DNA and integrated into a host's genome. Each type of virus has a preferred replication strategy that is dependent on the type of host cell infected, whether it be a eukaryotic or prokaryotic host cell. Thus, the virus has to adapt itself to varying conditions within the host. All viruses have similar problems, irrespective of how complex their replication processes are. The making of new virions (virus particles), the write-up of viral genes to make essential proteins, and the want for accurate genome replication [3].

Viruses have evolved a variety of tactics for getting around the restrictions placed on them by their host cells. They often do this by using special enzymes and factors to help with these processes, co-opting host translation and replication processes, or stealing host cell enzymes. This adaptation often results in the formation of specialized, virus-specific complexes that are crucial for the virus's life cycle [2].

Moreover, viral strategies directly affect how viral diseases affect humans, which is their pathology. The success of viruses as pathogens depends on their ability to reproduce within host cells, avoid the immune system, and transmit easily. The interaction between host immune defense strategies and viral replication has led to an ongoing evolutionary arms race in which viruses are constantly devising new means of escape from host immune surveillance and destruction. This chapter will look at the fascinating variety of viral reproduction mechanisms and will first overview the underlying principles of these systems before looking at specific reproduction strategies of different virus groups [1]. This section will explore how viruses overcome barriers to survive and propagate across various hosts and ecosystems. It will examine the different mechanisms of viral replication, detailing the stages involved and the strategies employed by various viral families. This will provide insights into how viruses interact with host systems, their molecular pathogenicity, and their evolution in diverse environments [3].

2. Common elements of viral replication cycles

The viral replication cycle consists of several different steps that together lead to the production of new infectious viral particles, called virions, by the virus. These activities help the virus to 'walk' along and infect new cells. The different types of viruses are diverse but they all share similar mechanisms of action like attachment, penetration, uncoating, macromolecular biosynthesis, assembly, and release. Throughout every stage of infection, the virus and its host interact intricately. It demonstrates many viral adaptations to take advantage of the host cell biology and evade its cellular defense system. This section goes over each step of the viral reproduction cycle in detail, paying particular emphasis to the intricate chemical processes and differences between different viral families [2].

2.1 Attachment and cell entry

When the virus comes into contact with the target host cell, a highly specialized attachment is made to start the replication cycle. Viruses use viral attachment proteins on their surface to bind to host cell receptors to achieve this. The receptors are usually the normal cellular proteins or carbohydrates that are involved in the host cell processes. Influenza viruses, for example, target sialic acid residues on the glycoproteins of respiratory epithelial cells. In contrast, HIV binds to the CD4 receptor on T cells, often requiring the coreceptors CCR5 or CXCR4. Tropism, which refers to the virus's preference for a particular type of infected cell or tissue, is a function of receptor binding specificity. Some viruses, such as the rabies virus, can infect many different types of hosts, but other viruses, such as the hepatitis B virus, are limited to specific infected tissues or species [2].

Tropism is determined by the presence of necessary coreceptors and receptor molecules on potential host cells. After attachment, the virus must enter the host cell. Proteins like gp41 in HIV or hemagglutinin (HA) in influenza viruses are fusion proteins. They help enveloped viruses like the herpes simplex virus (HSV) fuse their lipid envelope to a host cell's membrane. Non-enveloped viruses enter cells through receptor-mediated endocytosis. The virus uses the normal cellular mechanism, of forming clathrin-coated vesicles, to internalize into endosomes. When viruses enter host cells, they encounter additional obstacles, such as the endosomal compartments within the host cells [1, 2].

Many viruses cause changes in their attachment proteins due to the acidic effect within endosomes which help them release the core genome into the cytoplasm or nucleus. For example, the influenza virus has a pH-dependent conformational change in its HA protein, allowing the viral envelope and endosomal membrane to fuse [3].

2.2 Uncoating and genome release

In order to replicate, the viral DNA must be freed from its outer capsid after entering the host. Depending on the virus, this stage, known as uncoating, may occur at different cellular locations and involves the partial or complete disintegration of the viral capsid. Viruses, like that of poliovirus, inject their genome into the cytoplasm near the cell membrane, where uncoating occurs. Some viruses, such as herpesviruses, have different methods for entering the nucleus. Their capsid is transported there by microtubules, and the virus's DNA is released directly into the nucleus through the nuclear pore. Cell factors from host cells or particular environmental stimuli are often necessary for timing. At times, there are changes in the environment around the virus, like a drop in pH or enzyme activity, which cause uncoating. To separate the virus protein from its RNA segments, influenza viruses require endosomal acidification to activate their M2 ion channel. This allows RNA to leave and enter the cytoplasm for transcription and replication. The uncoating process is a series of carefully timed events that prevent early exposure of viral DNA, which could elicit recognition by innate immune sensors, such as Toll-like receptors, or be degraded by nucleases of the host [2, 3].

2.3 Macromolecular synthesis

The blueprint for viral replication and the creation of new virions is found in the uncoated genome. The kind of viral genome—single-stranded RNA (ssRNA), double-stranded RNA (dsRNA), single-stranded DNA (ssDNA), or double-stranded DNA (dsDNA)—determines the precise stages needed in macromolecular production [3].

2.4 Transcription and translation

The top priority of many viruses is viral mRNA. Adenoviruses and other DNA viruses usually transcribe viral mRNA in the nucleus by using host DNA-dependent RNA polymerase II. On the other hand, RNA viruses usually have their own specialized RdRps for synthesizing mRNA from their RNA genome in the cytoplasm.

- Viruses that are classified as positive-sense RNA viruses, including poliovirus, utilize the ribosomes of their host in the production of proteins by translating their genome [1].

- Negative-sense RNA viruses as rabies viruses need to make a positive-sense RNA strand first before they can translate [1].

- Retroviruses, including HIV, use the reverse transcriptase enzyme to turn their RNA genomes into DNA. The virus incorporates its DNA into the host genome, exploiting the host's transcriptional machinery [1].

2.5 Genome replication

To make offspring virions, the viral genome must replicate. DNA viruses often use the host's DNA polymerases to replicate in the nucleus. RNA viruses rely on RdRps encoded by specific viruses to assist in their cytoplasmic replication. Retroviruses utilize a particular two-step mechanism to integrate into the host genome after reverse transcription.

2.6 Protein synthesis and modification

Before functioning, viral proteins translated by host ribosomes often undergo posttranslational modifications like glycosylation or clipping. When a virus is first infecting a cell, it makes nonstructural proteins like RdRps or proteases but later on, it makes structural proteins like capsid and envelope proteins.

2.7 Assembly and maturation

The virus's DNA and proteins are built up to produce new virions after they have been made. Making capsids to pack viral genomes has been purposely given and structural proteins assemble spontaneously. Either in the cytoplasm, as seen in the case of poxviruses; or in the nucleus, herpesviruses. Maturation is an essential phase that ensures newly created virions become infectious. During this process, the virus or the host uses proteases to cleave precursor proteins. To make mature infectious particles, for instance, HIV needs a viral protease to cleave its Gag-Pol polyprotein into functional structural elements. Enveloped viruses acquire a lipid envelope when the host cell membrane wraps around the nucleocapsid during budding. The viral envelope glycoproteins help the virus attach to new host cells in the future [2].

2.8 Release and transmission

The last step of the replication cycle is the release of progeny virions. The enveloped viruses HIV and influenza typically make their egress from the host cell by budding, without adversely affecting the host cell. On one hand, adenoviruses and other unenveloped viruses commonly cause cell lysis which kills the host cell and releases virion. In order to infect new host cells, the virion must pass through the extracellular environment after its release. Viruses are transmitted in all possible ways, some by direct contact (like herpesvirus), some through respiratory droplets (like influenza), and some by vectors like mosquitoes (like dengue virus). Successful transmission defines the propagation of viral infections and often dictates the epidemiological consequence of a virus. The release and transmission stage also possess an essential battlefield for host immune defenses, like the role of neutralizing antibodies and immune surveillance systems. To ensure their survival and propagation, viruses often deploy strategies like immune evasion molecules and antigenic variation to dodge these defenses. Understanding the intricacies of each stage in the viral replication cycle has provided important insights into virology and the development of therapeutic strategies targeting particular stages of viral infection [4].

3. DNA virus replication

When the viruses enter the host cells, the replicative form is made from the DNA viral genome. Because the replication site varies and whether the genome is dsRNA or ssRNA, these viruses use a variety of replication strategies. A lot of DNA viruses use their host's cellular machinery. However, some of them, like the virus that replicates in the cytoplasm (where no host DNA polymerases are available), encode their own replication enzymes. This part of the chapter looks at the features and the site of replication of DNA viruses. It does so by looking at double-stranded and single-stranded DNA viruses as well as the function of host and viral enzymes. The presence of particular structural features, the circular or linear structure of the viral genome, and the virus's dependence on host or virally encoded enzymes are other factors that affect these tactics [4].

3.1 Rolling circle replication (RCR)

Some ssDNA viruses that use this mechanism include the geminiviruses and bacteriophage ΦX174. When a host cell transcribes viral ssDNA, it synthesizes a complementary strand. This creates a double-stranded replicative form (RF). The design of this RF is for more replication. Rep protein, which is a virally encoded endonuclease, acts by nicking one strand of the DNA at a specific site, creating a free 3′ hydroxyl (OH) group. DNA polymerase uses the 3' OH group as a starting point for elongation of the nicked strand. A "rolling" loop is created when the nicked strand unwinds and the intact strand serves as a template for DNA polymerase, which is producing new

DNA. The synthesis yields a long concatemer; that is, a single DNA strand consisting of many connected copies of the viral genome. The replication machinery keeps extending the DNA and sometimes forms complex structures, depending on which viral proteins and host factors are involved. The concatemer is properly packed into new virions when it is now long enough for subclasses of the enzymes to cut the concatemer into independent genomes at specific places. This very clever strategy allows viruses to rapidly produce large amounts of genetic material. RCR can generate a variety of genomes quickly and efficiently from a single circular template, which is the technique's main benefit [1, 3]. **Figure 1** gives a graphical representation of the RCR mechanism.

3.2 Rolling-hairpin replication (RHR)

Adeno-associated viruses (AAVs) and other linear ssDNA viruses use rolling-hairpin replication, a process that exploits the self-priming ability of the genome ends. A loop is produced by viral DNA folding back on itself within terminal hairpin structures. The structure provides a DNA polymerase with an available 3′ hydroxyl group. The polymerase starts by adding to the 3′ end and extending a complementary

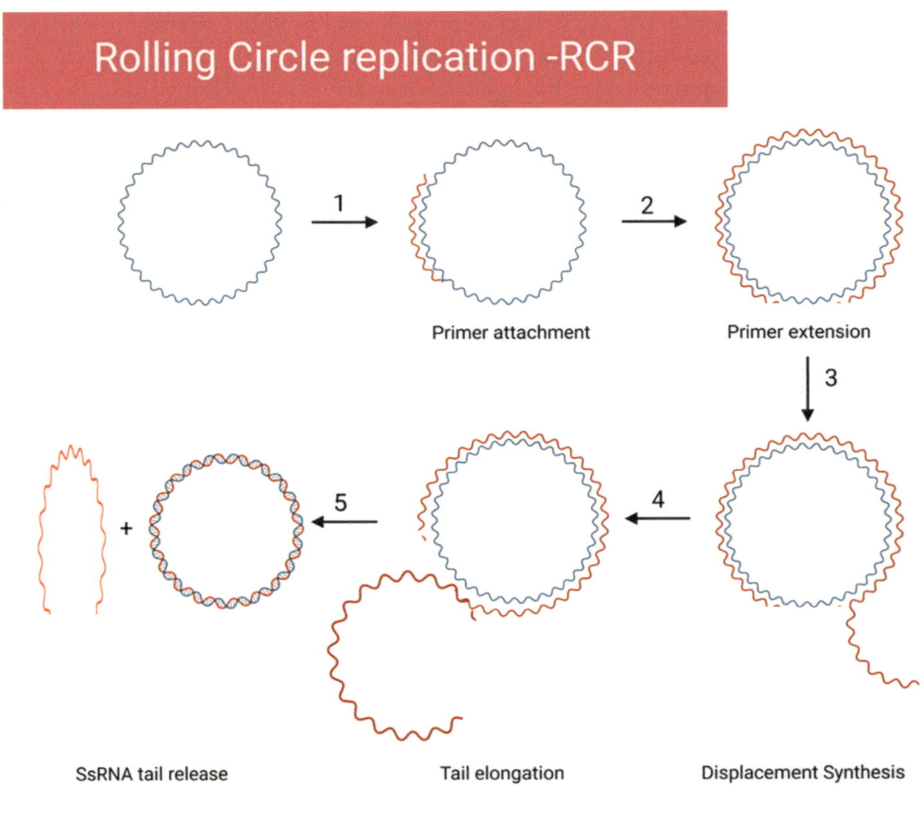

Figure 1.
(1) *A short complementary primer attaches to a circular ssRNA template.* (2) *It is extended by the template-directed primer extension process.* (3) *Upon attaining full length, the primer extends further by displacing the other end of itself from the initial point, resulting in an overhanging portion.* (4) *When the overhanging tail attains a length equal to that of the circular template, it breaks apart.* (5) *The separated tail becomes an open-ended ssRNA.*

strand; this displaces the original strand. To replicate further, a double-stranded intermediate is formed. After the double-stranded intermediate is formed, the displaced strand refolds to reestablish a hairpin configuration. This new hairpin will allow for further priming and so folding will ensure the ongoing activity of polymerase for DNA synthesis. The process is repeated until the entire genome is fully replicated. Specialized enzymes ensure genome replication is accurate and complete by resolving any secondary structures or junctions that form during this process. Linear viral genomes lend themselves best to this technique as a circular intermediary is not required. RHR allows linear ssDNA viruses to copy their genomes without needing circular intermediates.

Figure 2 shows the RHR process graphically [3, 5].

3.3 dsDNA bidirectional replication

This is the most common replication strategy among double-stranded DNA (dsDNA) viruses and it mimics the replication protocols of many biological organisms. Dedicated spots on viral genomes where the first replication steps happen are called origins of replication (ori). At these sites, the initiation complex assembles that

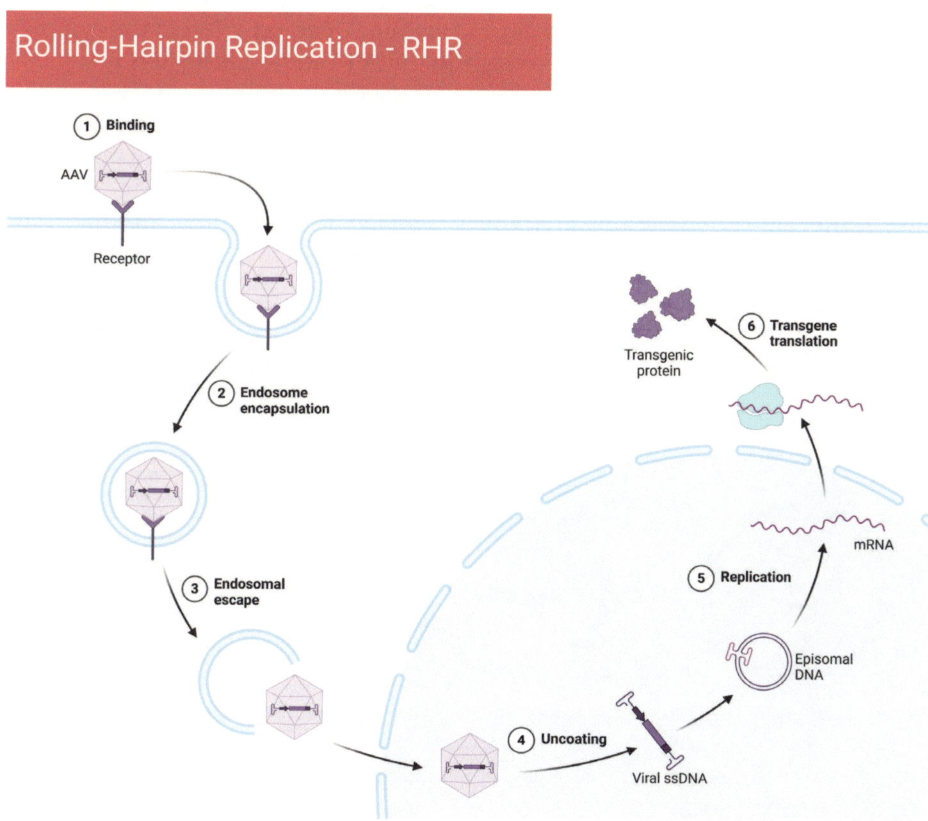

Figure 2.
It illustrates the rolling-hairpin replication mechanism of adeno-associated virus (AAV), highlighting the key steps involved in viral genome amplification. Initially, the single-stranded (+) DNA genome is encapsulated into the viral capsid and introduced into the host cell.

contain enzymes like topoisomerases to relieve supercoiling, helicases to unwind the DNA, and other accessory proteins. The Y-shaped point at which DNA replication occurs is known as a replication fork. DNA polymerase must have a short primer to start replication. Primase synthesizes a short RNA primer at the origin, providing the necessary 3' OH group. As DNA keeps getting made, little bubbles appear when replication starts at the origin and goes both ways. As the fork unwinds, the DNA polymerase travels in the same direction. As such, replication on the leading strand is continuous. Because the strands of DNA run in opposite directions, the lagging strand is synthesized discontinuously. The small Okazaki fragments are connected by ligase to form one strand. To ensure the replication of viral genomes effectively which is bidirectional in nature, it hijacks the machinery of host proteins. DNA replication can be bidirectional or monodirectional by the ease of its activity. **Figure 3** graphically illustrates this process [3, 1].

3.4 dsDNA (RT) transcription and replication

The hepatitis B virus and other retroviruses duplicate their circular dsDNA genomes using a more complicated process involving an RNA intermediate. The viral DNA is first moved to the nucleus where the host RNA polymerase converts it to pre-genomic RNA (pgRNA). Two functions of this RNA serve as a substrate for reverse transcription, and a template for protein translation. Once exported to the cytoplasm, the pgRNA is translated into reverse transcriptase (RT) and other structural elements of the virus. The pgRNA serves as a template for making a complimentary copy of DNA at the beginning of reverse transcription. After it is created, the RT enzyme has many activities, including DNA polymerase and RNase H activity, which permit the breakdown of the RNA strand of the RNA: DNA hybrid. A dsDNA genome forms by the use of the remainder, the single-stranded template for the synthesis of the second

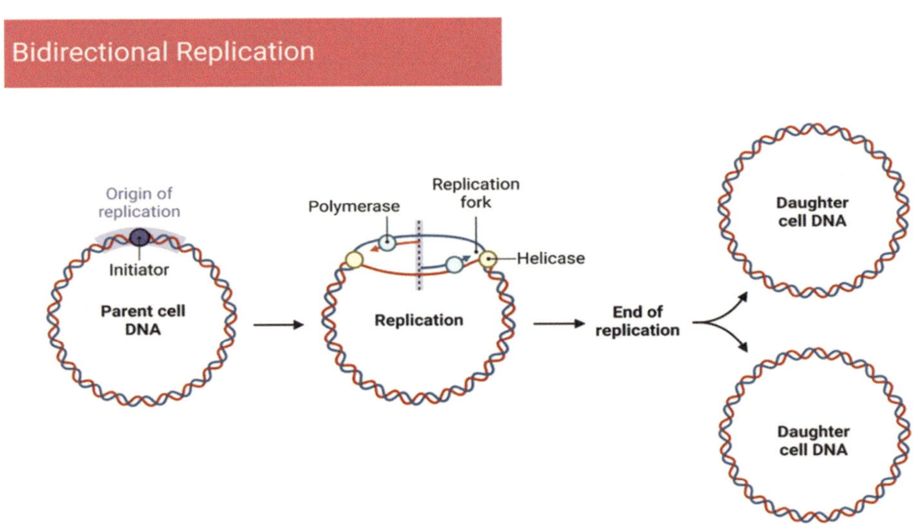

Figure 3.
This figure shows the initiation of bidirectional DNA replication, starting at the origin. DNA gyrase relieves supercoiling, followed by ssDNA binding proteins stabilizing the unwound DNA. RNA primase synthesizes a primer, and DNA polymerase begins replication in both directions from the origin.

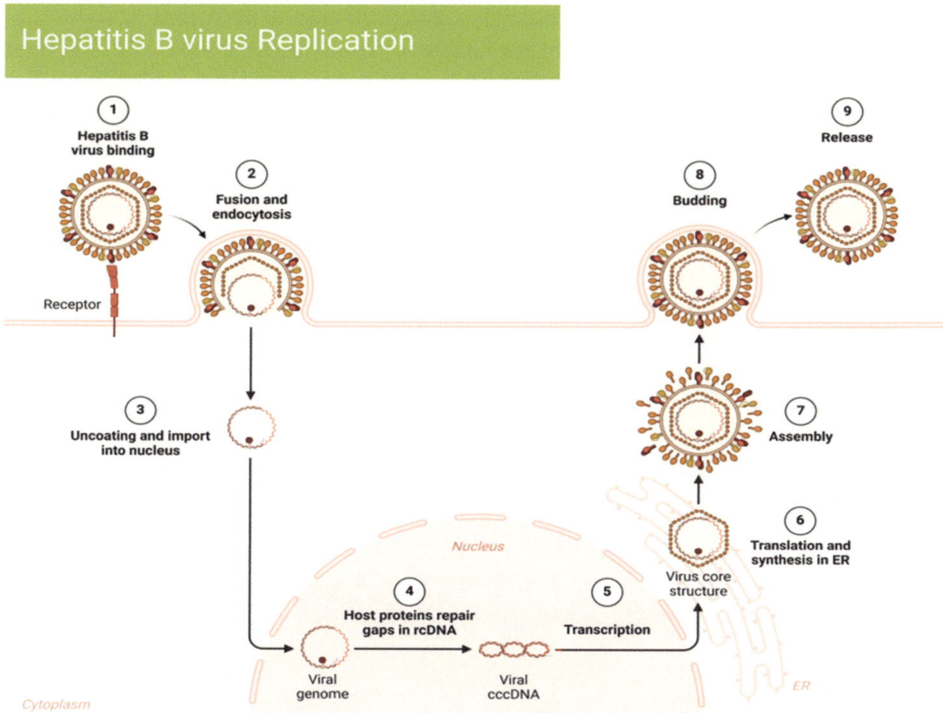

Figure 4.
This figure depicts the process of reverse transcription during viral replication. First, the reverse transcriptase (RT) binds to the epsilon (ε) region of the pgRNA and acts as a primer for replication (steps 1–2). It then synthesizes the minus-strand DNA (step 3), followed by degradation of the plus-strand by RNase H (step 4). Next, the DR-cap primer translocates (step 5) and initiates plus-strand DNA synthesis (step 6). Finally, the plus-strand DNA is translocated and the replication cycle is completed, resulting in the formation of the circular DNA (rcDNA) (steps 7–8).

DNA strand. The newly synthesized dsDNA may either enter the nucleus for subsequent transcription and replication cycles or be packaged into new viral particles. **Figure 4** in the book shows the process [5].

4. RNA virus replication

RNA viruses each use a different replication mechanism depending on the type of RNA genome, like double-stranded RNA, negative-sense single-stranded RNA, and positive-sense single-stranded RNA. The +ssRNA virus uses its viral genome as mRNA. Thus, it gets translated into proteins by the ribosomes of the host immediately. In a cell, a viral enzyme, called an RNA-dependent RNA polymerase (RdRps), first copies the RNA genome *via* the synthesis of a complementary negative-sense RNA strand. This negative-strand RNA will be then used to make additional positive-sense RNA genomes. In contrast, ssRNA viruses first use the RdRps that they carry in order to transcribe their genome into a complementary positive-sense RNA. This RNA is used to make copies of the genome and to make viral proteins (mRNA). To escape detection from the host immune response, dsRNA viruses transcribe mRNA from their double-stranded genome by the RdRps within the viral capsid. The synthesized mRNA is then used for making the genome and proteins [6].

Viruses like HIV have a genome which is a single strand of RNA that has a positive-sense and involves a DNA intermediate for replication. Because of this, they implicate a specialized strategy. The viral RNA is changed into DNA which is double-stranded by reverse transcriptase enzyme. The DNA merges with the host's genome. When the DNA mixes with the host, the virus uses the host's transcription system to make viral mRNA and genomic RNA. The variety of replication methods shows how flexible RNA viruses are and how much they rely on particular viral enzymes such as reverse transcriptase or RdRps. These enzymes are essential targets for antiviral treatments that try to stop viral replication and manage infection since they are not present in host cells [1]. **Figure 5** depicts the replication mechanism of different classes of RNA viruses.

4.1 Positive-strand RNA viruses

Positive-strand RNA viruses are advanced, complex, and diverse pathogens capable of sophisticated genome replication and other processes. Viruses have impressive

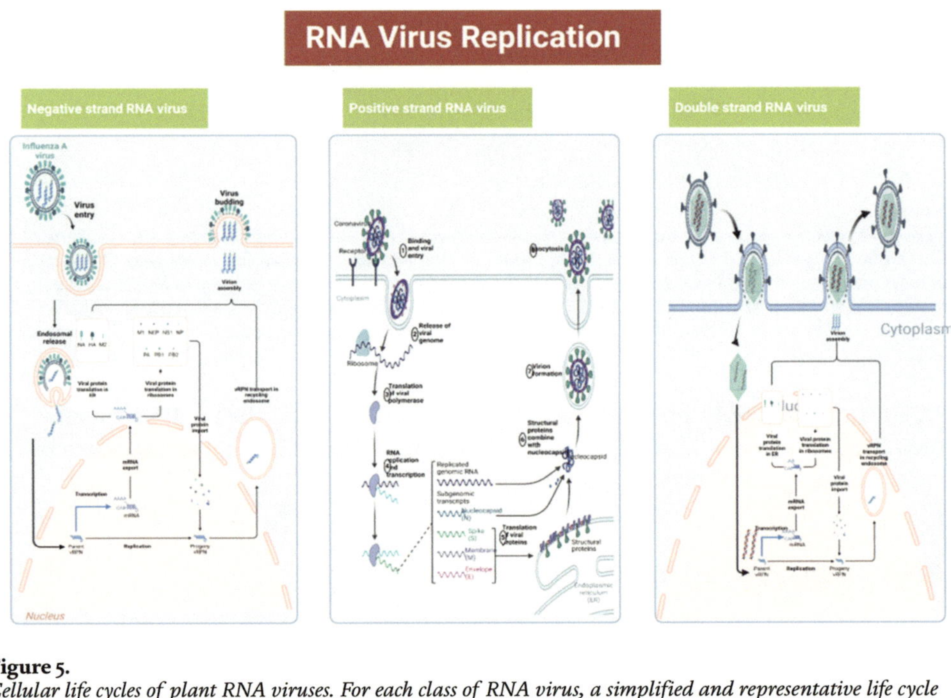

Figure 5.
Cellular life cycles of plant RNA viruses. For each class of RNA virus, a simplified and representative life cycle is shown. All three virus classes replicate exclusively through RNA intermediates in the cytoplasm. Nuclear trafficking of macromolecules during viral replication could not be ruled out. Virions are shown as black hexagons containing positive (+) and/or negative (−) RNA strands in red and green, respectively, and viral-RNA-dependent RNA polymerase (RdRp, blue circle). Other viral proteins are shown as filled circles of distinct colors. (a) The life cycle of (+) RNA viruses. The genomic RNA (gRNA) from virions is released into the cytoplasm. This (+) RNA, mRNA sense, is translated to produce several viral proteins including the viral RdRp. This polymerase copies the (+) strands into (−) strands that serve as templates for the synthesis of (+) strands that can be translated, replicated, or assembled in virion particles. (b) The life cycle of the majority of (−) RNA viruses. The gRNA is used as a template by the viral RdRp to generate (+) strand mRNAs that are released into the cytoplasm to be translated into viral proteins. The gRNA is also copied into full-length (+) strands that, in turn, serve as templates for (−) RNA synthesis. For members of the genus Nucleorhabdovirus*, replication occurs in the nucleus. (c) The life cycle of double-stranded RNA (dsRNA) viruses. Viral RdRp synthesizes and releases into the cytoplasm (+) strands that are first translated and then packaged to form immature virions. Virions mature by synthesizing (−) RNA and by the addition of other viral proteins.*

abilities and utilize host cell machinery in complex ways. Moreover, it helps them efficiently reproduce and avoid host immune responses. Flaviviruses, including clinically significant viruses such as dengue virus and West Nile virus, are known for their ability to adapt to different environments and hosts. The viral factories are made of reorganized host endoplasmic reticulum (ER) membranes. They create a compartment that protects viral RNA synthesis from the host antiviral response and achieves efficient replication [1, 7].

Coronaviruses, especially SARS-CoV-2, which made the headlines in 2020 as a result of a pandemic, use a similar approach as picornaviruses in making double-membrane vesicles (DMVs) from membranes of the host. These compartments are like complex and safe havens for viral RNA intermediate species where replication is well coordinated. Togaviruses, such as the Chikungunya virus, use different yet equally elegant strategies. The virus produces a comprehensive polyprotein that gets systematically cleaved into nonstructural proteins that are functional and essential for replication. This virus is such a good engineer on the molecular level that it uses a precisely regulated polyprotein to produce essential replication components [7].

Leviviridae bacteriophages incorporated tRNA-like structures at the 3′ end of their genomes as another amazing replication strategy. These structures help get that replicase complex in the right place. They ingeniously sew back on that lost terminal adenine which gets missing during negative-strand synthesis. Picornaviruses like poliovirus also have a sophisticated mechanism that uses the VPg. This is a small protein covalently attached to the genome's 5′ end. This protein performs several key functions, serving as a primer for RNA synthesis, and stabilizing the replication complex, thus enhancing the efficiency and fidelity of viral replication [1].

The different techniques of positive-strand RNA virus replication include those of caliciviruses and hepeviruses. They make use of structures from their host cells membranes as well as the breakdown of vesicles to replicate themselves. RNA synthesis among Alphaviruses, Flaviviruses, and Coronaviruses is temporally regulated and made more complex by strand-specific secondary structures and proper 3′ end sequences for the production of viral RNA [5].

4.2 Negative-strand RNA viruses

Viruses that have negative-strand RNA have developed an even more sophisticated way to separate replication from transcription. In other words, they are very clever with their genes. The mechanism utilized by the rhabdovirus (Vesicular Stomatitis Virus (VSV)) for stop-start transcription is a complicated one. It initiates from the 3′ end of the genome, transcribes a leader, terminates, and begins again at various gene junctions, adding a poly(A) tail to each mRNA. This is a very fine-tuned molecular mechanism for efficient viral gene expression [2].

Ebola and Marburg viruses, for instance, employ another sophisticated method. These filoviruses leverage a polymerase cofactor protein that balances the switch from transcription to replication. Viruses reproduce inside tightly regulated cytoplasmic viral factories which prevent immune detection of viral activities by the host cell. Viruses that belong to the group orthomyxovirus such as Influenza A, moreover, employ another unique mechanism of replicating in the cell nucleus and using the splicing machinery of their hosts for a more effective reproduction [3].

The bunyaviruses have non-segmented ambisense RNA, while paramyxoviruses produce capped and polyadenylated mRNAs within cytoplasmic inclusion bodies, and arenaviruses are segmented ambisense RNAs with internal genes encoded in opposite directions. These viruses have developed remarkably diverse mechanisms for protein synthesis and assembly, consistently relying on sophisticated interactions with host cellular components. The transition between mRNA production and the synthesis of antigenomic RNA relies on specific signals at the 3′ end, as well as regulatory proteins. The viral systems have amazing molecular engineering capabilities as this example shows [3].

4.3 RNA circles: Viroids, virusoids, and plant satellite viruses

Infectious agents that target plants include covalently closed circular RNA elements. These are interesting forms of agents. The Potato spindle tuber viroid, virusoids found in a range of plant viruses, and satellite viruses are remarkably simple to replicate. The rolling circle mechanism of these RNA circles creates many RNA strands, which are further processed into monomers to cause great agricultural harm despite their small size [6].

4.4 Viruses that use reverse transcriptase

Viruses that use reverse transcriptase are a group of complex pathogens that can change RNA into DNA and incorporate their genome into that of the host

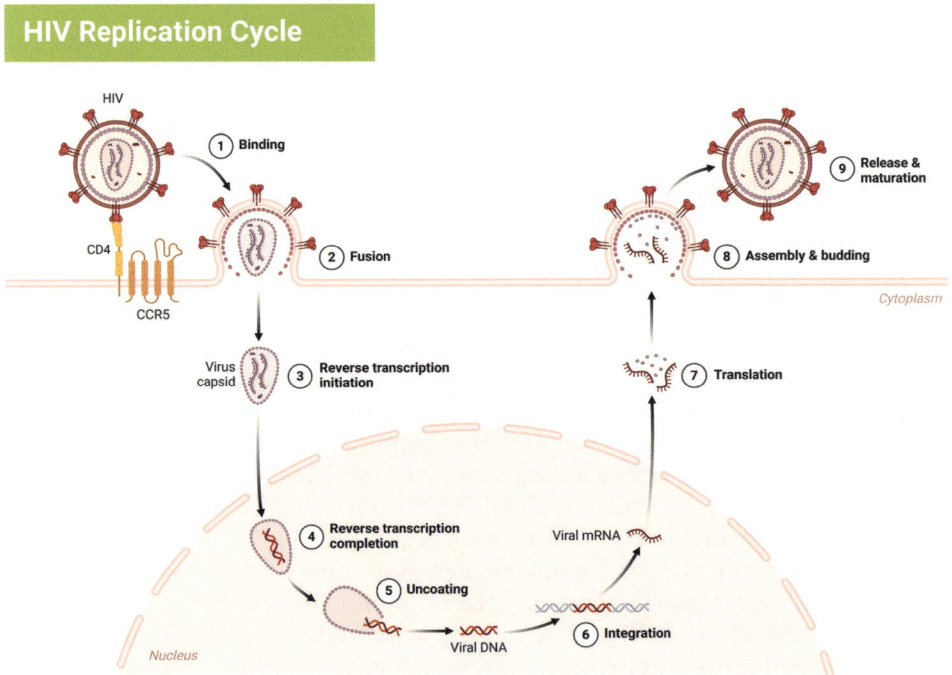

Figure 6.
This image illustrates the HIV replication cycle, which begins with the virus binding to CD4 receptors and co-receptor CCR5 on the host cell (step 1). After fusion with the host membrane (step 2), the virus releases its RNA into the cytoplasm. Reverse transcription converts the viral RNA into DNA (steps 3 and 4), which is then uncoated and integrated into the host's genome (steps 5 and 6). Viral mRNA is transcribed and translated (step 7) to produce viral proteins. These proteins assemble into new virions, which bud from the host cell and mature to become infectious (steps 8 and 9).

permanently. The strategy V viruses (retroviruses) use to replicate is illustrated by HIV. This is a complex multi-step process (see figure) where first, reverse transcriptase makes complementary DNA. Secondly, RNase H degrades the other RNA strand. Finally, double-stranded DNA forms. The viral integrase is important for correctly integrating viral material into the host genetic material [1, 6]. **Figure 6** depicts the replication mechanism of HIV RNA viruses.

Hepadnaviruses and cauliflower mosaic virus (CaMV) are also capable of reverse transcription, having been shown to exist integrated and episomally in their hosts. The replication methods face significant challenges from host restriction factors like APOBEC3 proteins and SAMHD1, which try to induce mutations and limit the availability of nucleotides. Even with all these great cell defenses, reverse transcriptase is still an important molecule that helps viruses to stay alive and replicate. Even now, retrotransposons are still changing our DNA a whole lot [2].

5. Conclusion

Viral replication strategies are very diverse, which shows these viruses are very smart to survive and replicating using the machinery of the host cells. Even though they are simple, viruses have finely tuned mechanisms of a particular type that are tailor-made to the virus's DNA, RNA, or reverse-transcribing RNA to suit their medium. The cycle of virus replication includes stages such as attachment and uncoating, genome replication, assembly, and release. These stages of virus replication show that viruses and a host have fine-tuning.

The use of rolling circle and rolling-hairpin replication in DNA viruses and RNA-dependent RNA polymerases in RNA viruses, as well as reverse transcriptase in retroviruses, highlights the importance of understanding how these mechanisms work and their evolutionary origin. Viruses are masters of molecular adaptation. They can make special structures for replicating their genetic material. They can adapt to the immune evasion strategy of the host.

Furthermore, the ways viruses reproduce can teach mathematicians valuable lessons in the future. By studying how viruses act in hosts and how they replicate, we can figure out how to stop the virus. For example, RNA viruses depend on special enzymes which are the RdRps. Additionally, the integration direct by a number of retroviruses provides a specific stage that is druggable. Reverse transcriptase inhibitors used for the treatment of HIV are an example.

To sum up, the examination of how viruses duplicate sheds great light on how flexible these things are. It shows they can not only survive different ecological pressures but also affect the evolution of their hosts. Research in the future will uncover more novel replication and therapeutic options in this space.

Author details

Dheeraj Kumar
The Indus Hospital and Health Network, Karachi, Pakistan

*Address all correspondence to: dheerajutradi7@gmail.com

References

[1] Hershey HV, Taylor MW. Strategy of Replication of the Viral Genome. US: Springer eBooks; 1987. pp. 47-98. DOI: 10.1007/978-1-4684-5350-8_3

[2] Louten J. Virus replication. Essential Human Virology. 2016;**1**:49-70. DOI: 10.1016/B978-0-12-800947-5.00004-1

[3] Rampersad S, Tennant P. Replication and expression strategies of viruses. In: Viruses. Basel, Switzerland: MDPI: 2018. pp. 55-82. DOI: 10.1016/b978-0-12-811257-1.00003-6

[4] Deng H, Cao H, Wang Y, Li J, Dai J, Li LF, et al. Viral replication organelles: The highly complex and programmed replication machinery. Frontiers in Microbiology. 2024;**15**:1450060. DOI: 10.3389/fmicb.2024.1450060

[5] Staufer O, Gantner G, Platzman I, Tanner K, Berger I, Spatz JP. Bottom-up assembly of viral replication cycles. Nature Communications. 2022;**13**(1):1-10. DOI: 10.1038/s41467-022-33661-7

[6] Finke S, Conzelmann KK. Replication strategies of rabies virus. Virus Research. 2005;**111**(2):120-131. DOI: 10.1016/j.virusres.2005.04.004

[7] Leyssen P, De Clercq E, Neyts J. Molecular strategies to inhibit the replication of RNA viruses. Antiviral Research. 2008;**78**(1):9-25. DOI: 10.1016/j.antiviral.2008.01.004

Chapter 3

Hepatitis B Virus (HBV) Integration into the Host Genome and Molecular Mechanisms

Sisi Chen, Xin Yan, Hao Kang, Yunrui Ru, Wenyan Wu, Davgadorj Chantsalmaa and Yan Yan

Abstract

Hepatitis B Virus (HBV)—infected host cells include more complex replication strategies and procedures. By delving into the replication strategy of the HBV, scientists can better understand its life cycle and infection mechanism, providing a theoretical basis for developing effective antiviral treatments. The replication strategy of the HBV involves multiple steps, including genome reverse transcription, DNA synthesis, and assembly of viral particles, each of which is a potential drug target. The integration of HBV has a significant impact on its life cycle and can promote the long-term survival and transmission of the virus in the host. The integration of the HBV may interfere with the normal function of host genes, lead to changes in cell signaling pathways, and may even promote tumorigenesis. Through high-throughput sequencing technology and bioinformatics analysis, scientists were able to pinpoint the integration site of the HBV in the host genome, providing a basis for subsequent research. Studies have shown that specific integration sites of the HBV are associated with the severity of liver disease, which offers new ideas for early diagnosis and treatment of the disease.

Keywords: hepatitis B virus (HBV), life cycle, integration, detection, mechanism

1. Introduction

Hepatitis B Virus (HBV), a double-stranded DNA virus, can cause life-long chronic infection, resulting in liver fibrosis, cirrhosis, and hepatocellular carcinoma (HCC) [1]. HBV is distinguished by its pronounced tissue and species specificity and can cause a distinctive genomic structure and an asymmetric replication mechanism [2]. Electron microscopy allows for the visualization of various viral particles in infectious serum, including infectious virions and subviral particles. Infectious viral particles, known as Dane particles, have a spherical double-layer structure of 42–44 nm, containing an icosahedral core particle assembled by HBV core antigen (HBcAg). The core particle mainly contains relaxed circular DNA (rcDNA) and the covalently bound viral polymerase [2]. This rcDNA is the HBV genome, with a length of approximately 3.2 kb, slightly varying among different genotypes, forming the nucleocapsid with the core protein. The DNA of HBV is enveloped by a layer of capsid

IntechOpen

proteins, which bear hepatitis B core antigen (HBcAg) and hepatitis B e antigen (HBeAg). Beyond the capsid proteins, there is an envelope protein that embeds varying proportions of large, medium, and small hepatitis B surface antigens (large/medium/small HBsAg). These surface antigens are proteins that are acquired during the budding of the virus from the endoplasmic reticulum (ER) [3].

In Dane particles, the negative strand of the viral rcDNA exists at its full length, carrying complete genetic information, and is covalently linked to the HBV polymerase through a phosphotyrosine bond. However, the positive strand of the viral rcDNA is approximately two-thirds the length of its genome [1, 4], with a short RNA oligonucleotide from the pregenomic (pgRNA) remaining at the 5′ end in a covalently bound form, known as the residual RNA primer. Additionally, the negative DNA strand possesses a minor redundant segment of 8–9 nucleotides at both the 5′ and 3′ end, designated as the R region. These residual and redundant structural elements are crucial for the replication of the virus [2, 5]. HBV pgRNA is reverse-transcribed within the nucleocapsid, resulting in the development of a rcDNA genome or a double-stranded linear DNA (dslDNA). DslDNA molecules can result in viral integration into the host cell genome. Even though this step is not necessary for viral replication, the exact mechanisms and functions of HBV integration are undergoing intensive investigation. Including the exact purpose, timing, molecular pathways involved, the dependence on viral and host factors, the viral antigens expressed form, integrated forms, and their possible contribution to viral persistence [6].

2. The life cycle of HBV

The entry of HBV into cells is a highly specific and regulated process that involves receptor recognition, endocytosis, and transport to the nucleus [4]. The initial stage of HBV infection of hepatocytes involves the binding of viral particles to the hepatocyte surface (**Figure 1**). Initially, HBV undergoes low-affinity binding and high-affinity binding with the hepatocyte. After undergoing HBV high-affinity binding with sodium taurocholate cotransporting polypeptide (NTCP), there is a process known as adsorption. The HBV-NTCP complex dynamically transfers from the cell surface to the membrane vesicles, achieving viral internalization [7, 8]. The receptor mediates the entry of viral DNA into the cell nucleus and paves the way for subsequent steps of viral replication and infection. The released rcDNA genome into the nucleoplasm is then repaired by host cell enzymes into a stable covalently closed circular DNA (cccDNA) and forms a minichromosome structure within the nucleus. cccDNA serves as a template for subsequent viral gene expression and replication, transcribed by host cell RNA polymerase II to produce viral mRNA and pgRNA, a step that is crucial for the persistent infection and replication of the virus. On the one hand, the transcribed viral mRNA is translated into viral proteins, such as HBx protein, which further stimulates the transcription of cccDNA and promotes viral replication; on the other hand, the transcribed pgRNA combines with the viral polymerase (P protein) to form a pgRNA-pol protein complex, which is packaged into newly formed nucleocapsids, reverse transcribed into new rcDNA within the nucleus. The rcDNA is either redelivered to the nucleus to form a cccDNA pool or re-encapsulated with viral envelopes, forming mature viral particles and further released from the cell through the multivesicular body pathway [8].

Understanding this mechanism is crucial for developing therapeutic strategies aimed at preventing HBV infection and managing liver diseases associated with the

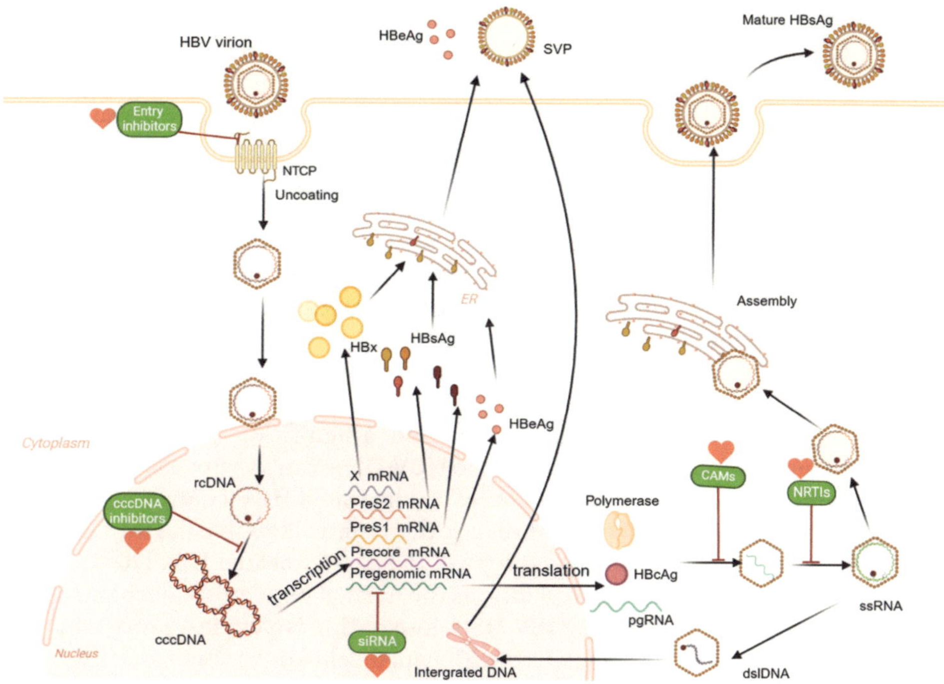

Figure 1.
The HBV replication cycle. Subsequently, HBV releases its duplex, and the relaxed-circular DNA (rcDNA) genome is transported into the nucleus. Then rcDNA genome is converted into covalently closed circular DNA (cccDNA) in the nucleus, which acts as a transcriptional template for pregenomic RNA (pgRNA) and mRNA, allowing HBV infection to continue within the organism. The pgRNA is encapsulated together with HBV polymerase (Pol) protein into a nucleocapsid composed of HBV core proteins. Pol-mediated reverse transcription of pgRNA occurs in the nucleocapsid, leading to the formation of (1) rcDNA or (2) double-stranded linear DNA (dslDNA). rcDNA can either be enveloped and secreted as virions or to migrate to the nucleus and replenish the intranuclear cccDNA reservoir. Conversely, there is a small proportion of nucleocapsids that contain dslDNA, which not only can be released as enveloped virions but also can be transported to the nucleus, contributing to the further replenishment of the cccDNA pool via homologous recombination. Notably, the dslDNA that has entered the nucleus can also integrate into the host cell genome by exploiting cellular repair mechanisms, such as non-homologous or microhomology-mediated end joining. HBV virions enter hepatocytes in the endocytic form by highly specific binding to the receptors on the surface of hepatocytes, Sodium Taurocholate Cotransporting Peptide (NTCP), followed by uncoating before they enter into the cytoplasm. CAM: capsid assembly modulator; NRTI: nucleoside reverse transcriptase inhibitors.

virus. The replication of HBV involves several steps, including reverse transcription of the genome, DNA synthesis, and assembly of viral particles, each of which represents a potential drug target [9]. By thoroughly investigating the replication strategies of HBV, scientists can gain a deeper understanding of its life cycle and infection mechanisms, thereby providing a solid theoretical foundation for developing effective antiviral therapies.

3. HBV DNA integration

HBV DNA integration is defined as the process where the viral DNA inserts itself into the host's genomic DNA [10]. Integration occurs somewhat rarely, at a rate of 1 per 10^3–10^4 cells [1, 11]. The integration sites of HBV in the host genome are widely distributed, and the study found that 7513 HBV integration breakpoints are spread throughout the human genome [12]. About 36.9% of the breakpoints are preferentially distributed in a specific region of the HBV genome, including relevant coding sequences. Moreover, compared with expectations, more breakpoints are observed in the X protein and core protein. The research results support the view that HBV breakpoints in these regions may promote the formation of HBV-human fusion genes to initiate the occurrence of liver cancer [12]. The lengths of integrated fragments vary, ranging from 28 to 3215 bp, and long fragments are relatively more frequent. At the same time, HBV integration at some sites can lead to changes in the structure of the host genome, such as the appearance of sequence duplications or inverted insertions of complementary sequences, indicating that HBV integration may induce instability in the host genome [12, 13]. The clinical study showed that the HBV integrated inter-chromosomal translocation appears in one-third of patients [14].

This integration is not a random occurrence but a significant event with far-reaching consequences. Once integrated, the HBV DNA can disrupt the normal functioning of host genes [15]. The presence of integrated HBV contributes to the instability of the chromosomal structure in patients and allows for the transcription and translation of viral proteins, including HBsAg and truncated HBx [16–18]. This disruption can lead to genomic instability, as the normal regulatory mechanisms of the host genome are perturbed. HBV DNA integration is a critical process in the pathogenesis of HBV and its association with hepatocellular carcinoma (HCC) [19]. Integrated HBV DNA can activate known oncogenes and other growth-promoting genes, cause chromosomal instability, and may induce epigenetic changes, thereby promoting tumor growth [20, 21]. The integration of HBV DNA into the host genome was once considered a byproduct of the viral life cycle but is now recognized as a significant contributor to HBV-induced liver diseases, including HCC and the persistence of hepatitis D virus (HDV) [22]. The integrated HBV DNA can also have an impact on the replication and persistence of the virus itself. It may interact with the viral replication machinery in ways that either enhance or inhibit replication. Additionally, the presence of integrated HBV DNA in the host genome can contribute to the long-term persistence of the virus within the host, making it more difficult to eliminate HBV from the body [23].

Although its early occurrence in infection strongly suggests a crucial role in these processes, the exact molecular and cellular mechanisms remain to be fully deciphered and understood. Accurate identification of HBV integration sites is crucial for understanding the full extent of the virus's impact on the host genome. The advent of next-generation sequencing (NGS) technologies has revolutionized the identification of HBV integration sites. NGS allows for high-throughput sequencing of large amounts of DNA, enabling the detection of even rare integration events. It can provide detailed information about the sequence context of the integration sites, including the surrounding host genome sequences and any associated genomic rearrangements [24]. The integration sites can be further analyzed to understand the pathways and networks affected by HBV integration, providing insights into the molecular mechanisms of carcinogenesis [24]. The integration of HBV DNA into the human genome can lead to significant restructuring of the genome architecture in HCC, promoting major chromosomal rearrangements and alterations in oncogenic drivers [15, 19]. This emphasizes the importance of understanding and identifying the HBV integration sites for the diagnosis, treatment, and prognosis of chronic HBV infection and HCC patients [25].

4. The mechanisms of HBV DNA integration

Firstly, HBV integration events are less frequent during the acute phase of infection, but the frequency of integration significantly increases with prolonged infection, especially in patients with chronic infection where the virus replicates over the long term [22]. This suggests that the cell cycle and the state of viral replication have a significant impact on the activity of integrase. Secondly, the replication or integration is also regulated by the virus's own proteins. The HBV X protein (HBx) can activate the preS1 promoter (Sp1), promoting the expression of Histone acetyltransferase 1 (HAT1), forming a positive feedback regulation pattern that aids in HBV replication [26]. The HAT1/Cancer-associated fibroblasts 1 (CAF-1) signaling pathway can facilitate the assembly of histones 3/4 on HBV cccDNA, thereby participating in the acetylation modification of histones on the HBV cccDNA minichromosome, affecting the production of integration [26]. The integrated HBV sequence can act as an enhancer, upregulating the transcription level of telomerase reverse transcriptase (TERT) through cis-activation, which may be related to the host immune response and the production of inflammatory factors [19]. Lastly, the host immune system also affects the procession of integration. HBV integration can upregulate the RNA expression levels of TERT, which is not only related to the integration site of HBV but also closely related to the integrated HBV sequence. The integrated HBV sequence can act as an enhancer, upregulating the transcription level of TERT through cis-activation, which may be related to the host immune response and the production of inflammatory factors [19]. In summary, the regulatory mechanisms of integrase are complex, involving the interaction between the host cell environment, the virus's own proteins, and the host immune system. These factors collectively influence the integration progress.

Hepadnaviral DNA also occurs at the time of chromosome double-strand break repair. It depends on the production of viral double-stranded linear DNA ends and the expression of I-Scel [27]. The major mechanisms of double-strand break repair in mammalian cells include non-homologous end joining and homologous recombination [28].

5. Innovative application of HBV DNA integration detection

5.1 High-throughput sequencing technology

Application and optimization of HBV sequence capture-sequencing technology help to increase the detection sensitivity and specificity of integration events [29]. Including hybrid capture sequencing, the HBV probe capture-sequencing technology, designing specific hybridization probes to enrich HBV integration fragments, has been widely used [29]. Therefore, these methods can significantly increase detection sensitivity, reduce host genome background interference, provide comprehensive coverage of HBV subtype sequences, and be able to detect HBV integration events more accurately [12]. It has been proven that some of them are able to discover many low-frequency integration sites, providing the possibility for in-depth research on the relationship between HBV integration and diseases. In this technology, probe design covers multiple HBV subtypes (A - H), ensuring comprehensiveness and accuracy of detection, which helps study the integration characteristics of different genotypes of HBV and their roles in diseases [12].

5.2 Whole genome sequencing (WGS) and transcriptome sequencing (RNA-Seq) collaborative analysis

WGS provides panoramic information on HBV integration sites, and RNA-Seq focuses on changes at the transcript level as a complementarity sequencing technology. It has been proven that combine the two can help to deeply understand the impact of HBV integration on gene expression regulation and reveal the molecular mechanism of HBV integration in the occurrence and development of diseases from multiple dimensions [30]. However, traditional Sanger sequencing can be used to verify the results of high-throughput sequencing. By performing Sanger sequencing on some integration sites, the accuracy of the results was ensured, the reliability of the study was improved, and false positive or false negative results were reduced [12].

5.3 Optimization of integration site identification algorithm

Innovation in the bioinformatics analysis process can help precisely determine the location of integration breakpoints. Qiao et al. [31] developed specific scripts and algorithms. First, sequencing data can be map to the HBV genome. Valid reads are retained according to strict alignment criteria. Then, it is mapped to the human genome. The characteristics of chimeric reads and paired-end reads are analyzed. Through operations such as merging breakpoints within a certain range, the location of integration breakpoints is accurately determined, improving the accuracy of detecting integration sites.

The development of functional annotation and pathway analysis tools helps analyze the multi-level functional annotation of HBV integration-related genes. Ding D et al. used Gene Ontology (GO) analysis to deeply understand the functions of HBV-targeted genes from multiple levels and found their enrichment in aspects such as cAMP metabolism and immune response; the DAVID Functional Annotation tool analyzed gene protein domains and revealed the enrichment of specific domains in genes related to HBV integration; KEGG pathway analysis mapped integrated genes to biological pathways to understand the impact of HBV integration on cell signal transduction and physiological processes, revealing the relationship between HBV integration and diseases from a systems biology perspective [12, 21].

6. Research prospect

6.1 Improvement of disease diagnosis and prognosis assessment

High-throughput sequencing technology can detect the information including HBV integration sites, viral load, and gene expression profiles, which is helpful in developing more accurate and sensitive diagnostic methods for hepatitis B and related diseases. Through the analysis of a large number of clinical samples, establishing a diagnostic model based on molecular markers can achieve early diagnosis and monitoring of disease progression. For example, detecting the expression level of specific HBV integration target genes (ITGs) can be used as an indicator for early diagnosis and prognosis evaluation of liver cancer [12, 13, 32].

Single-cell sequencing technology can reveal the dynamic changes of cells in the tumor microenvironment and provide more comprehensive and accurate information for prognosis evaluation of diseases such as Diffuse Large B-cell lymphoma (DLBCL). By monitoring the changes in tumor cells and immune cell subsets before and after treatment, it is possible to predict the treatment response and recurrence risk of patients and adjust the treatment plan in time to improve the survival rate and quality of life of patients [33].

6.2 Reveal the mechanism of virus-host interaction

Deeply understanding the interaction between HBV, HDV, and host cells in integration, including gene expression and signal pathways, will help to know the mechanisms of gene regulatory network during HBV integration after infection. It will help to develop more accurate antiviral treatment strategies, inhibiting virus replication and transmission by targeting key nodes of virus-host interaction. It has been shown that the distribution of HBV integration sites is related to the expression changes of host genes. Further exploring the impact of these changes on the physiological functions of cells can provide new targets for intervening in HBV infection [32, 34].

In addition, single-cell sequencing technology has great potential to reveal cellular heterogeneity in the tumor microenvironment. For diseases such as DLBCL, it can more accurately depict different subsets of tumor cells and immune cells and their functional states, which helps to deeply understand the intercellular interaction network in the process of tumor occurrence and development and provides a basis for personalized treatment. For example, according to the characteristics of cell subsets in the tumor microenvironment of different patients, targeted immunotherapy regimens are formulated to improve treatment effects [33, 35].

6.3 Develop new treatment strategies

Based on gene editing technologies such as clustered regularly interspaced short palindromic repeats (CRISPR)/CRISPER-associated (Cas) systems, it is expected to develop treatment methods directly targeting the HBV genome, such as precisely excising integrated HBV DNA or correcting HBV-related gene mutations to achieve a functional cure for hepatitis B. At the same time, using gene editing technology to modify immune cells can enhance their ability to recognize and kill HBV-infected cells, providing new means for immunotherapy.

Constructed cell lines such as HepG2BD can be used as in vitro models for screening and evaluating new antiviral drugs against HBV. By simulating the *in vivo* virus infection and replication process, it is possible to test the efficacy and safety of drugs quickly and efficiently, accelerating the process of new drug development. In addition, these cell lines can also be used to study virus resistance mechanisms and provide clues for solving the problem of drug resistance in antiviral treatment [36, 37].

Acknowledgements

This work was supported by the Top Talent Support Program for Young and Middle-Aged People of Wuxi Health Committee (BJ2023092), and the National Natural Science Foundation of China (81701550).

Conflict of interest

The authors declare no conflict of interest.

Author details

Sisi Chen[1,2†], Xin Yan[1,2†], Hao Kang[1], Yunrui Ru[1], Wenyan Wu[1], Davgadorj Chantsalmaa[1] and Yan Yan[1,2*]

1 Clinical Medical Research Center, The Fifth People's Hospital of Wuxi (Wuxi Infectious Disease Hospital), Affiliated Hospital of Jiangnan University, Wuxi, China

2 Wuxi School of Medicine, Jiangnan University, Wuxi, China

*Address all correspondence to: yanyan198134@hotmail.com

† There are the same contributions.

References

[1] Tu T, Budzinska MA, Vondran FWR, Shackel NA, Urban S. Hepatitis B virus DNA integration occurs early in the viral life cycle in an in vitro infection model via sodium taurocholate cotransporting polypeptide-dependent uptake of enveloped virus particles. Journal of Virology. 2018;**92**:e02007-e02017. DOI: 10.1128/JVI.02007-17

[2] Nassal M. HBV cccDNA: Viral persistence reservoir and key obstacle for a cure of chronic hepatitis B. Gut. 2015;**64**:1972-1984. DOI: 10.1136/gutjnl-2015-309809

[3] Hoffmann J, Boehm C, Himmelsbach K, Donnerhak C, Roettger H, Weiss TS, et al. Identification of alpha-taxilin as an essential factor for the life cycle of hepatitis B virus. Journal of Hepatology. 2013;**59**:934-941. DOI: 10.1016/j.jhep.2013.06.020

[4] Summers J. The replication cycle of hepatitis B viruses. Cancer. 1988;**61**:1957-1962. DOI: 10.1002/1097-0142(19880515)61:10<1957::aid-cncr2820611004>3.0.co;2-0

[5] Zhao Q, Chang J, Rijnbrand R, Lam AM, Sofia MJ, Cuconati A, et al. Pregenomic RNA launch hepatitis B virus replication system facilitates the mechanistic study of antiviral agents and drug-resistant variants on covalently closed circular DNA synthesis. Journal of Virology. 2022;**96**:e0115022. DOI: 10.1128/jvi.01150-22

[6] Tu T, Zhang H, Urban S. Hepatitis B virus DNA integration: In vitro models for investigating viral pathogenesis and persistence. Viruses. 2021;**13**:180. DOI: 10.3390/v13020180

[7] Herrscher C, Roingeard P, Blanchard E. Hepatitis B virus entry into cells. Cells. 2020;**9**:1486. DOI: 10.3390/cells9061486

[8] Niklasch M, Zimmermann P, Nassal M. The hepatitis B virus nucleocapsid-dynamic compartment for infectious virus production and new antiviral target. Biomedicine. 2021;**9**:1577. DOI: 3390/biomedicines9111577

[9] Schulze A, Gripon P, Urban S. Hepatitis B virus infection initiates with a large surface protein-dependent binding to heparan sulfate proteoglycans. Hepatology. 2007;**46**:1759-1768. DOI: 10.1002/hep.21896

[10] Howell J, Seaman C, Wallace J, Xiao Y, Scott N, Davies J, et al. Pathway to global elimination of hepatitis B: HBV cure is just the first step. Hepatology. 2023;**78**:976-990. DOI: 10.1097/hep.0000000000000430

[11] Yang W, Summers J. Integration of hepadnavirus DNA in infected liver: Evidence for a linear precursor. Journal of Virology. 1999;**73**:9710-9717. DOI: 10.1128/JVI.73.12.9710-9717

[12] Yang L, Ye S, Zhao X, Ji L, Zhang Y, Zhou P, et al. Molecular characterization of HBV DNA integration in patients with hepatitis and hepatocellular carcinoma. Journal of Cancer. 2018;**9**:3225-3235. DOI: 10.7150/jca.26052

[13] Shen-Gunther J, Easley A. HPV, HBV, and HIV-1 viral integration site mapping: A streamlined workflow from NGS to genomic insights of carcinogenesis. Viruses. 2024;**16**:975. DOI: 10.3390/v16060975

[14] van Buuren N, Ramirez R, Soulette C, Suri V, Han D, May L, et al.

Targeted long-read sequencing reveals clonally expanded HBV-associated chromosomal translocations in patients with chronic hepatitis B. JHEP Reports: Innovation in Hepatology. 2022;**4**:100449. DOI: 10.1016/j.jhepr.2022.100449

[15] Sung W-K, Zheng H, Li S, Chen R, Liu X, Li Y, et al. Genome-wide survey of recurrent HBV integration in hepatocellular carcinoma. Nature Genetics. 2012;**44**:765-769. DOI: 10.1038/ng.2295

[16] Wooddell CI, Yuen M-F, Chan HL-Y, Gish RG, Locarnini SA, Chavez D, et al. RNAi-based treatment of chronically infected patients and chimpanzees reveals that integrated hepatitis B virus DNA is a source of HBsAg. Science Translational Medicine. 2017;**9**:eaan0241. DOI: 10.1126/scitranslmed.aan0241

[17] Hu B, Wang R, Fu J, Su M, Du M, Liu Y, et al. Integration of hepatitis B virus S gene impacts on hepatitis B surface antigen levels in patients with antiviral therapy. Journal of Gastroenterology and Hepatology. 2018;**33**:1389-1396. DOI: 10.1111/jgh.14075

[18] Gu Z, Jiang Q, Abulaiti A, Chen X, Li M, Gao N, et al. Hepatitis B virus enhancer 1 activates preS1 and preS2 promoters of integrated HBV DNA impairing HBsAg secretion. JHEP Reports: Innovation in Hepatology. 2024;**6**:101144. DOI: 10.1016/j.jhepr.2024.101144

[19] Sze KM, Ho DW, Chiu YT, Tsui YM, Chan LK, Lee JM, et al. Hepatitis B virus-telomerase reverse transcriptase promoter integration harnesses host ELF4, resulting in telomerase reverse transcriptase gene transcription in hepatocellular carcinoma. Hepatology. 2021;**73**:23-40. DOI: 10.1002/hep.31231

[20] Zhao K, Liu A, Xia Y. Insights into hepatitis B virus DNA integration-55 years after virus discovery. Innovation (Camb). 2020;**1**:100034. DOI: 10.1016/j.xinn.2020.100034

[21] Ding D, Lou X, Hua D, Yu W, Li L, Wang J, et al. Recurrent targeted genes of hepatitis B virus in the liver cancer genomes identified by a next-generation sequencing-based approach. PLoS Genetetics. 2012;**8**:e1003065. DOI: 10.1371/journal.pgen.1003065

[22] Zoulim F, Chen P-J, Dandri M, Kennedy PT, Seeger C. Hepatitis B virus DNA integration: Implications for diagnostics, therapy, and outcome. Journal of Hepatology. 2024;**81**:1087-1099. DOI: 10.1016/j.jhep.2024.06.037

[23] Tu T, Budzinska M, Shackel N, Urban S. HBV DNA integration: Molecular mechanisms and clinical implications. Viruses. 2017;**9**:75. DOI: 10.3390/v9040075

[24] Cui X, Li Y, Xu H, Sun Y, Jiang S, Li W. Characteristics of hepatitis B virus integration and mechanism of inducing chromosome translocation. Npj. Genomic Medicine. 2023;**8**:11. DOI: 10.1038/s41525-023-00355-y

[25] Álvarez EG, Demeulemeester J, Otero P, Jolly C, García-Souto D, Pequeño-Valtierra A, et al. Aberrant integration of hepatitis B virus DNA promotes major restructuring of human hepatocellular carcinoma genome architecture. Nature Communications. 2021;**12**:6910. DOI: 10.1038/s41467-021-26805-8

[26] Yang G, Feng J, Liu Y, Zhao M, Yuan Y, Yuan H, et al. HAT1 signaling confers to assembly and epigenetic regulation of HBV cccDNA minichromosome. Theranostics. 2019;**9**:7345-7358. DOI: 10.7150/thno.37173

[27] Bill CA, Summers J. Genomic DNA double-strand breaks are targets for hepadnaviral DNA integration. Proceedings of the National Academy of Sciences of the United States of America. 2004;**101**:11135-11140. DOI: 10.1073/pnas.0403925101

[28] Scully R, Panday A, Elango R, Willis NA. DNA double-strand break repair-pathway choice in somatic mammalian cells. Nature Reviews Molecular Cell Biology. 2019;**20**:698-714. DOI: 10.1038/s41580-019-0152-0

[29] Fukano K, Wakae K, Nao N, Saito M, Tsubota A, Toyoshima T, et al. A versatile method to profile hepatitis B virus DNA integration. Hepatology Communications. 2023;**7**:e0328. DOI: 10.1097/HC9.0000000000000328

[30] Budzinska MA, Shackel NA, Urban S, Tu T. Cellular genomic sites of hepatitis B virus DNA integration. Genes (Basel). 2018;**9**:365. DOI: 10.3390/genes9070365

[31] Qiao L, Li C, Lin W, He X, Mi J, Tong Y, et al. ViroISDC: A method for calling integration sites of hepatitis B virus based on feature encoding. BMC Bioinformatics. 2024;**25**:177. DOI: 10.1186/s12859-024-05763-0

[32] Ringlander J, Stromberg LG, Stenback JB, Andersson ME, Abrahamsson S, Skoglund C, et al. Enrichment reveals extensive integration of hepatitis B virus DNA in hepatitis delta virus-infected patients. The Journal of Infectious Diseases. 2024;**230**:e684-e693. DOI: 10.1093/infdis/jiae045

[33] Ye X, Wang L, Nie M, Wang Y, Dong S, Ren W, et al. A single-cell atlas of diffuse large B cell lymphoma. Cell Reports. 2022;**39**:110713. DOI: 10.1016/j.celrep.2022.110713

[34] Li X, Zhang J, Yang Z, Kang J, Jiang S, Zhang T, et al. The function of targeted host genes determines the oncogenicity of HBV integration in hepatocellular carcinoma. Journal of Hepatology. 2014;**60**:975-984. DOI: 10.1016/j.jhep.2013.12.014

[35] Shi J, Li Q, Li J, Zhou J, Zhang X, Wang S, et al. Single-cell RNA sequencing reveals the spatial heterogeneity and functional alteration of endothelial cells in chronic hepatitis B infection. International Journal of Molecular Sciences. 2024;**25**:7016. DOI: 10.3390/ijms25137016

[36] Li J, Liu S, Zang Q, Yang R, Zhao Y, He Y. Current trends and advances in antiviral therapy for chronic hepatitis B. Chinese Medical Journal (English). 2024;**137**:2821-2832. DOI: 10.1097/CM9.0000000000003178

[37] Feitelson MA, Arzumanyan A, Spector I, Medhat A. Hepatitis B x (HBx) as a component of a functional cure for chronic hepatitis B. Biomedicine. 2022;**10**:2210. DOI: 10.3390/biomedicines10092210

Chapter 4

Morbillivirus Replication and Immune Evasion: Implications for Vaccine Design

Ashok Kumar, Ram Kumar, Anil Gattani and Sanju Mandal

Abstract

Morbillivirus, a genus within the Paramyxoviridae family, includes critical human and veterinary pathogens such as the measles virus, canine distemper virus (CDV), rinderpest virus (RPV), and peste des petits ruminants virus (PPRV). The understanding of morbillivirus replication, which encompasses viral attachment, fusion, transcription, replication, and virion assembly, is fundamental for advancing therapeutic interventions. The complex interplay between proviral and antiviral cellular signaling pathways, including those regulating innate immune responses and apoptosis, is central to both viral pathogenesis and host immune evasion. Morbilliviruses deploy various immune evasion strategies, such as the suppression of type I interferon responses, to establish persistent infections. Delineating these molecular mechanisms is critical for optimizing vaccine development and designing antiviral therapeutics, particularly in response to emerging viral strains. This chapter explores morbillivirus replication dynamics, immune evasion tactics, key signaling pathways, and recent advancements in vaccine and antiviral therapeutic strategies for managing these pathogens in human and veterinary populations.

Keywords: morbillivirus, viral replication, immune evasion, signaling pathways, vaccine development

1. Introduction

Morbilliviruses belong to the order *Mononegavirales*, the family *Paramyxoviridae*, and the subfamily *Paramyxovirinae*, known as pleomorphic, enclosed, negative-sense, single-stranded RNA viruses that replicate intracytoplasmically [1, 2]. Measles virus (MV), rinderpest virus (RPV), peste des petits ruminants virus (PPRV), canine distemper virus (CDV), cetacean morbillivirus, phocine distemper virus, and feline morbillivirus are the seven known members of the genus morbillivirus [3]. Both humans and animals infected with the morbillivirus experience severe immunosuppression [4], although those who survive often acquire lifetime immunity [5]. It is thought that different morbillivirus prototypes exhibit cross-protection. Viruses require more than just raw ingredients for nucleic acid and protein synthesis to spread successfully within their host. While research has focused on particular host components used by viruses, there is still a lack of quantitative functional insights for all host factors needed for viral reproduction. Viruses employ the host cell's machinery to replicate themselves, creating "viral factories" through protein-RNA and protein-protein interactions [5]. Viral pathogenicity and host range are determined by molecular interactions with cellular components. High-throughput sequencing and proteomics technologies have discovered hundreds of host components essential for virus replication, providing insights into potential targets for antiviral medication development [6].

2. Genome organization

Pleomorphic, enclosed, negative-sense, single-stranded viruses that replicate intracytoplasmically are known as paramyxoviruses. In animals, this family causes multisystemic, neurological, and respiratory disorders. A single strand of RNA, somewhat less than 16 kbp in length, makes up the genomes of morbilliviruses. The six structural proteins—the nucleocapsid (N), the phospho (P), the matrix (M), the fusion (F), the hemagglutinin (H), and the large (L) proteins—are encoded by the six contiguous, nonoverlapping transcription units into which they are arranged [7]. The latter is the viral RNA-dependent RNA polymerase. Their 3′ (leader) and 5′ (trailer) terminal extremities include highly conserved regions that function as transcription and replication promoters **Figure 1**. Sequences extending into the untranslated area at the beginning of the N gene open reading frame (ORF) and the untranslated region at the end of the L gene ORF are examples of full promoter elements. All

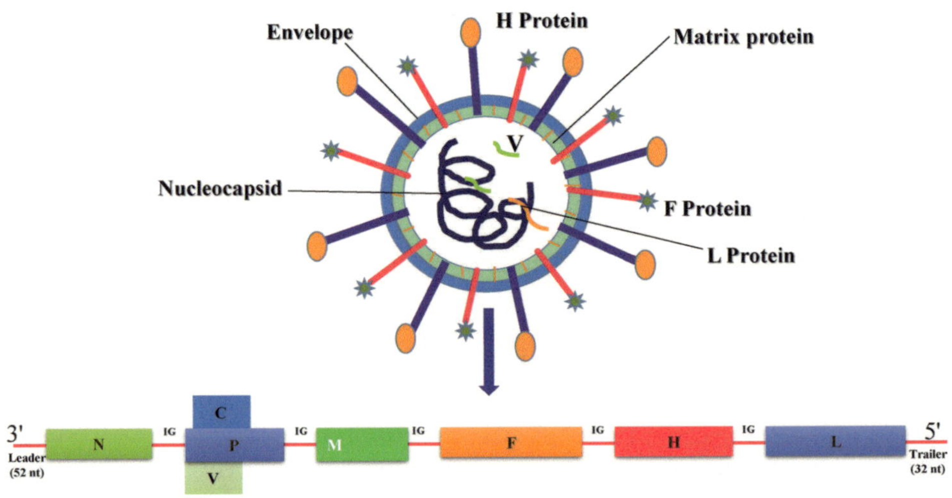

Figure 1.
Schematic diagram of a Morbillivirus, Genome arrangement of virions are enveloped and pleomorphic in shape which varies in size from 150 to 700 nm (Mean size 500nm). The virions contain a negative-strand RNA genome enclosed in a ribonucleoprotein (RNP) core. The genomic RNA is packaged by nucleoprotein (N) to form nucleocapsid along with phosphoprotein (P) and large protein (L). The virus genome is ~16kb in length (15948 nts) which consists of six structural (N, P, M, F, H and L) and two non-structural (V and C) proteins. At the 3′ and 5′ ends, there are untranslated regions of 52 nt and 32 nucleotide, respectively. IG = Intergenic Region, N = Nucleocapsid Protein, P= Phosphoprotein, M = Matrix Protein, F = Fusion Protein, H = Hemagglutinin Protein and L = Large Protein (Polymerase).

of the cis-acting signals required for initial transcription and the creation of a complete positive-sense RNA genome copy, which is necessary for the synthesis of new genome RNA, are found in these locations. Each mRNA transcription unit has semiconserved start-stop sequence motifs at the beginning and end: (UCCU/C) at the beginning of the transcription and a sequence rich in U residues at the end that indicates the polyadenylation of the mRNAs. An intergenic triplet, often GAA, sits between the end of one transcription unit and the beginning of the next. Upstream mRNA termination is necessary for downstream mRNA synthesis. The RNP core, the transcription/replication unit of the virus, is made up of the N, P, and L proteins as well as the genomic RNA. During the budding process, the host cell produces a lipid envelope that contains the F and H glycoproteins [8]. The two components that make up the budded virion are brought together by the nonglycosylated M's interaction with the cytoplasmic domains of the membrane-associated F and H proteins as well as the nucleocapsid RNPs that are created in the cytoplasm during replication. For viral budding to be effective, the M protein is required. Morbilliviruses produce two nonstructural proteins (C and V), which are encoded in the P gene transcription unit. Ribosomes that scan past the first AUG codon and begin at the second, which is located approximately 20 nt downstream, translate the first of these, the C protein. This protein has no antigenic connection to the P protein and is in a separate reading frame [9]. By adding a nontemplated G residue to around 50% of the P mRNAs, alternative transcription of an mRNA from the P transcription unit yields the second nonstructural protein, the V protein. About halfway up the P protein ORF, the additional Gs are inserted in a particular, highly conserved region called the editing site (5′ UUAAAAAGGG[G]CACAG). Since manmade transcription systems do not exhibit this so-called editing process, it is a characteristic of the viral polymerase. The V protein, a chimeric protein made up of the N-terminus of the P protein and a new, shorter C-terminus rich in cysteine residues obtained from the template sequence in the third reading frame, is produced when this mRNA is translated. Because its coding region is situated before the editing point in P, the V mRNA can also translate the C protein [10].

In addition to regulating transcription and replication, the nonstructural proteins help viruses evade the host's innate immune responses. Morbilliviruses must have a genome length that is divisible by six (the "rule of six"), just like certain other paramyxoviruses [11]. The reason for this need is that each N protein monomer binds to precisely 6 nt, and effective transcription and/or replication are only possible if the complete RNA genome is encapsulated by the N protein. For MV, RPV, and CDV, reverse genetics methods have been developed. This makes it possible for a virus to be "rescued" from a copy of its genome, which can then be altered to create viral mutants [12]. These may be used to investigate the molecular underpinnings of host range and pathogenicity, as well as to ascertain the roles of different proteins and sequence patterns.

3. Virus replication

3.1 Infection and virus attachment

The virus's pathogenesis and host susceptibility are heavily influenced by the initial phase of infection, which involves attaching to host cells and delivering the nucleocapsid into the cytoplasm. The PPRV initially interacts with the host by attaching to cellular receptors *via* its attachment protein, the HN protein [13]. Morbilliviruses effectively reproduce in lymphocytes after first targeting lymphoid tissues. The molecule that signals lymphocyte activation (SLAM), the main cellular receptor for morbilliviruses is also known as CD150 **Figure 2**. The viruses have great lymphoid cell tropism since it is only expressed in immune cells [14]. Signaling molecule for lymphocyte activation by screening a cDNA library obtained from B95a cells, which are extremely permissive for MV [15, 16], discovered SLAM for the first time. When a single clone of marmoset B (B95a) cells was transfected, 293 T cells which are

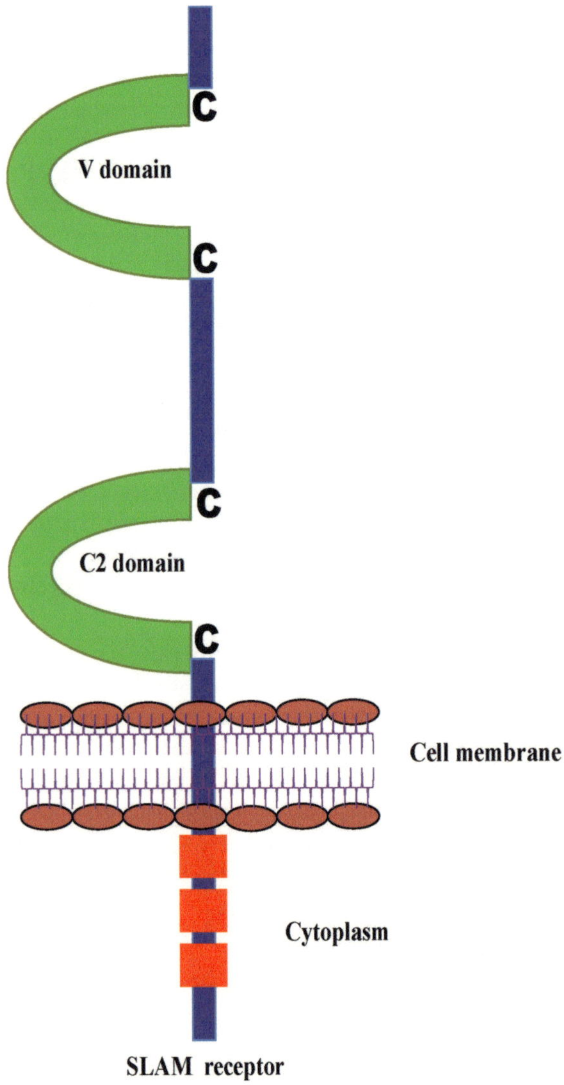

Figure 2.
Schematic diagram of SLAM receptor molecule: *The extracellular domain is composed of a variable (V) and a constant (C2) Ig-like repeat. Its cytoplasmic domain contains three tyrosine residues (red block) that are surrounded by SH2 domain binding sequences. The morbillivirus H protein binds to the V domain on the target cells, which triggers viral infection.*

normally nonsusceptible became susceptible to the vesicular stomatitis virus pseudotype that carries the MV H protein. Lymphocytes, monocytes, dendritic cells, and macrophages are the main cells that express SLAMs [17]. Since SLAMs control T cell activation and can also control the activities of natural killer and dendritic cells, they play a wide role in the modulation of both innate and acquired immune responses [17, 18]. Every morbillivirus attaches itself to SLAM's V domain. The adapter molecules connected to the cytoplasmic tail of SLAM are the SLAM-associated protein (SAP) or EWS/FLI-1-activated transcript 2. Another SLAM molecule in the nearby cells may form an association with the extracellular domain of SLAM. When SLAM engages, it binds to SAP and initiates downstream signaling that causes T helper 2 cytokines to be upregulated [16]. SLAM interacts with the following MV-H protein residues: I194, D505, D507, Y529, D530, T531, R533, H536, Y553, and P554 [19]. A morbillivirus's complete pathogenicity requires SLAM-mediated cell entrance. The recombinant SLAM-blind lapinized strain of RPV is highly virulent in rabbits and has similar pathogenicity to virulent RPV in cattle, making it a suitable model for studying RPV's *in vivo* pathogenicity [20].

A virus's host range and tissue tropism are determined by its cellular receptors. SLAMs found in humans, dogs, cattle, and goats serve as shared receptors for measles virus MV, CDV, RPV, and PPRV [21, 22] found that monkey cells expressing goat SLAM are more sensitive to PPRV separation from clinical material than those expressing cow SLAM. B95a cells are commonly used to isolate MV, CDV, RPV, and PPRV due to their high surface expression of SLAM [15]. Morbilliviruses infect epithelial cells of the intestines, liver, lungs, trachea, bronchial tubes, oral cavity, esophagus, pharynx, and bladder without SLAMs, indicating the presence of alternate cellular receptors. *In vitro* studies have shown that morbillivirus can cause cytopathology and virus generation in SLAM-negative cell types, including epithelial and neuronal cells.

Paramyxoviruses initially infect the upper respiratory tract epithelium from the luminal side before spreading to lymphatic cells [23]. A novel model suggests that wild-type MV spreads throughout the body by infecting SLAM-expressing lymphatic cells, rather than requiring initial virus amplification in respiratory epithelial cells [16, 23]. Infecting rhesus monkeys with an epithelial receptor-blind MV, which does not recognize epithelial receptors but maintains SLAM-dependent entrance, resulted in virulence but no virus shedding, indicating the importance of additional cellular receptors in virus dispersion [24]. Two different research groups identified a novel morbillivirus receptor, PVRL4 (Nectin-4), expressed on epithelial (i.e., I456, L464, L482, P497, Y541, and Y5430) [24, 25]. The Nectin family proteins have three Ig-like loops (V and two C2-type domains) in their extracellular domain **Figure 3**. Nectin-4 is the sole member of the Nectin family that acts as an epithelial cell receptor [13, 26–28]. The other three members do not. After systemic infection, infected lymphocytes and dendritic cells may spread the virus to epithelial cells *via* Nectin-4 on the basolateral side. Morbilliviruses can be found in endothelial and neuronal cells, in addition to lymphocytes and epithelial cells [20]. According to Sato, MV, and CDV cause persistent encephalitis due to their significant neural cell tropism and lack of expression of SLAM and Nectin-4. Morbillivirus cell entrance can occur without SLAM, CD46, or Nectin-4 in several cell lines [23, 29]. This book chapter suggests the presence of other receptors. According to Fujita, heparin-like glycosaminoglycans, cellular cyclophilin B, and CD147 may act as morbillivirus receptors in cells. Both SLAM and Nectin-4 have been linked to PPRV entrance into host cells. While SLAM

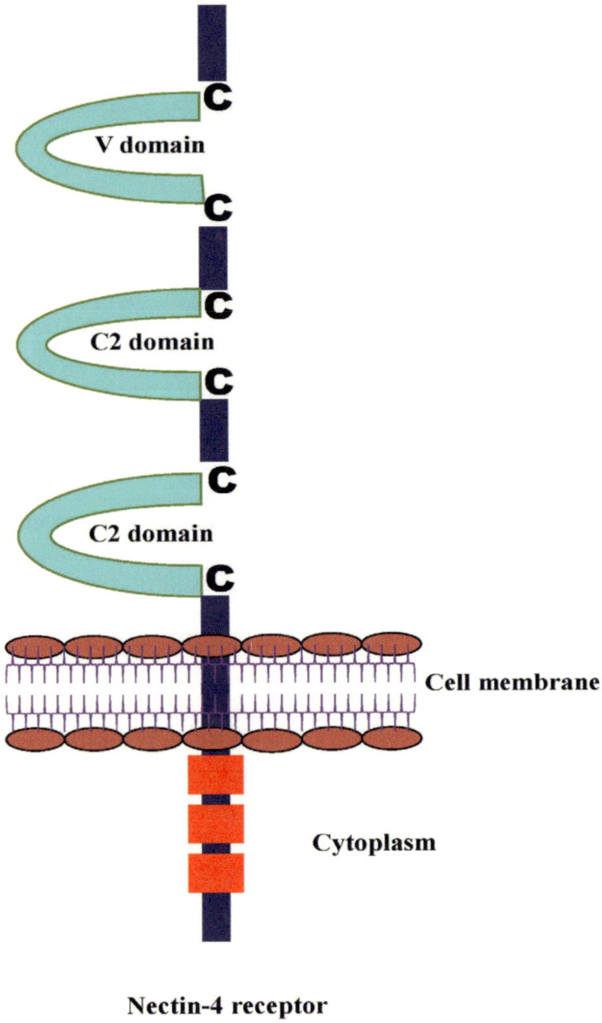

Figure 3.
Schematic diagram of Nectin-4 receptor molecule: *The extracellular domain is composed of a variable (V) and a two constant (C2) Ig-like repeat. Its cytoplasmic domain contains three tyrosine residues (red block) that are surrounded by SH2 domain binding sequences. The morbillivirus H protein binds to the V domain on the target cells, which triggers viral infection.*

is crucial for initial engagement, Nectin-4 acts as an exit receptor to spread the virus throughout the body and promote its amplification and release through various secretions [13, 30, 31].

3.2 Virus entry

Paramyxoviruses typically cause lytic infection in cell cultures. However, high-titer virus yields require adaptation through the selection of mutants that can replicate in the *in-vitro* system. Syncytia are common in paramyxovirus infections in non-polarized cell cultures, but less so in polarized systems. Syncytia are also present in some, but not all, paramyxovirus infections in animals [32, 33]. Paramyxovirus infections are characterized by acidophilic cytoplasmic inclusions made of ribonucleoprotein structures. Morbilliviruses, on the other hand, produce acidophilic intranuclear inclusions made of nuclear elements and N protein. Paramyxoviruses with the HN protein exhibit hemadsorption. The paramyxovirus fusion (F) proteins mediate viral penetration by fusing the virions' envelope with the host cell plasma membrane, which happens at neutral pH. *Morbillivirus* entry principally depends on the H and F proteins [32] that closely associate to facilitate membrane fusion at a neutral pH. The result of the fusion reaction is that the nucleocapsid is delivered to the cytoplasm. Later in infection, the F proteins produced at the plasma membrane of infected cells can facilitate fusion with nearby cells to generate syncytia (giant cell development), a cytopathic impact that can lead to tissue necrosis *in vivo* and may also be a virus dissemination mechanism. Sialic acid, an acyl derivative of neuraminic acid, is found in both glycoproteins and lipids (sialoglycolipids or gangliosides). Gangliosides operate as both an attachment factor and a receptor for the Sendai virus [34]. The cellular receptor for the morbillivirus measles virus is the cell surface protein CD150SLAM, and the cellular receptor for pneumoviruses, though not proven, appears to involve binding to glycosaminoglycans containing the disaccharide heparan sulfate and chondroitin sulfate B. The M protein shell in the viral particle is thought to have multiple interactions with the nucleocapsid [35]. When the viral envelope fuses with the cell's plasma membrane and the nucleocapsid is released into the cytoplasm, a mechanism must exist to disrupt the M-N connections.

3.3 Virus RNA replication and transcription

Morbillivirus RNA replication and transcription occur within the cytoplasm. Infecting virions include RNA-dependent RNA polymerase (RdRp), which stimulates the synthesis of mRNA and complementary RNA. Transcription begins when RdRp binds to the GP on genomic RNA [7]. The transcriptional units (coding sequence and noncoding surrounding regions) are produced in a start-stop' manner. The RdRp can access a downstream transcriptional unit only when the preceding unit is fully synthesized. RdRp can detach from the template (IG) and restart transcription at GP, allowing for control over the amount of protein generated. The N protein is highly transcribed due to its proximity to the GP. The L protein with the lowest transcription rate is positioned farthest from the GP. Paramyxoviruses transcribe specific mRNA species as naked RNA. The virus-encoded polymerase caps the 5′ end and polyadenylates the 3′ end, making the RNA stable and efficient for translation by host ribosomes [7]. The mRNA transcript contains polyadenylation signals (UUUU) before each IG region, as reported by Munir et al. [36]. Unlike other viral transcripts, the morbillivirus P gene generates three distinct proteins: P, a structural protein, and C and V, nonstructural proteins. According to Munir, the first initiation codon creates the P protein, while the second start codon produces the C protein *via* an alternate reading frame. The absence of the first AUG in the ideal Kozak consensus sequence (A/GXXAUGG) hinders protein synthesis efficiency [37]. Cotranslational editing adds one or more G residues to the P mRNA at a conserved editing location (3 ′-AAUUUUUCCCGUGUC-5 ′) to produce the mRNA for the V protein [38]. The RdRp changes to produce complementary RNA (antigenome RNA) at some point after the mRNA is synthesized. cRNA and the N protein are linked, much as genomic RNA. One theory holds that the RdRp function is switched from mRNA to cRNA synthesis due to the accumulation of unassembled N protein in the cytoplasm [39], while another theory postulates the existence of two distinct forms of RdRp, one for transcription and one for replication [40].

3.4 Virus assembly and release

New paramyxovirus particles are created when the surface glycoproteins, M protein, and ribonucleoproteins (RNPs) assemble at the plasma membrane and then bud. Not much is known about how the morbillivirus assembles and releases. Paramyxovirus assembly and release are significantly influenced by the M protein. By binding with nucleocapsid at virus assembly sites, it acts as an adapter to connect the structural elements of the virions (viral glycoproteins and RNPs) with cellular membranes. It also promotes the incorporation of genomic RNA into budding virions. While M is the primary protein in charge of paramyxovirus assembly and release, additional viral proteins including H, and a number of host variables have also been suggested, along with F and C. Viral components agglomerate at distinct locations on cellular membranes, followed by host cell membrane protrusion, in the precise and intricate process of viral protein assembly. Lipid rafts can serve as platforms for virus assembly because they are abundant in sphingolipids and cholesterol, which have a rigid, structured structure with little flexibility [10, 41]. Instead of being equally distributed across the cell surface, RNA virus envelope glycoproteins are grouped within the membrane microdomains of lipid rafts to create the budding nucleation sites [10]. The raft microdomains are the specific target of paramyxovirus glycoproteins. In certain viruses, both glycoproteins can attach to the rafts, while in others, only the F protein—not the H protein—has the inherent capacity to be integrated into membrane rafts [42]. Other viral components, including the N [43] and M proteins [44], can also attach to the lipid raft microdomains in addition to the glycoproteins. Multiple membrane microdomains can coalesce as viral components accumulate at cell membranes, allowing viruses to construct their own platforms for assembly [10]. In addition to serving as locations for assembly, the raft domains enhance the freshly generated paramyxovirus particles' contagiousness. Paramyxovirus particles form when all structural components of the virus are assembled at specific sites on membranes. These particles bud and pinch off to spread the infection to new cells/hosts [45]. Some paramyxoviruses, including MV and SV, require lipid rafts for assembly but not for budding.

3.5 Virus budding

Enveloped viruses create membrane protrusions, followed by membrane scission and liberation from infected cells. In addition to viral-host protein interactions, viral proteins interact with membrane lipids to induce membrane curvature and fission [46]. Paramyxovirus budding is primarily driven by the M protein, which binds and oligomerizes beneath the plasma membrane. This causes membrane distortion and curvature development. Harrison et al. [47] and Takimoto and Portner [48] have identified multiple methods for paramyxovirus budding. The L domain of paramyxovirus M proteins, also known as P[T/S]AP, PPxY, or YxxL, plays a role in late budding. The L domain interacts with the Endosomal Sorting Complex Required for Transport (ESCRT) system proteins and promotes membrane fission, resulting in the release of virus particles from the plasma membrane. Paramyxovirus budding can occur through ESCRT-dependent [49] or independent [50] pathways. SV budding is well characterized among paramyxoviruses [51]. The ability of the SV-F protein to form a bud depends on a TYTLE motif in the protein's cytoplasmic tail [52], indicating that this motif is required for efficient binding. The cytoskeleton may play a role in paramyxovirus budding, as evidenced by the presence of actin associated with SV and mutations in the actin-binding domain of the SV-F protein that reduces SV-like particle production. El Najjar et al. [45] found that the cytoplasmic tail domains of glycoproteins have a role in the budding process of paramyxoviruses, in addition to other exocytic components. Glycoprotein clustering in lipid raft microdomains pulls on the plasma membrane, causing initial deformation and further elongation by M protein oligomerization [53] to promote virus budding. Although the intrinsic glycoprotein targets the basolateral surface of polarized epithelial cells, the M protein directs budding to the apical surface. M's loss of apical targeting and surface [41, 54, 55], promotes cell-cell fusion at the expense of virus generation.

4. Immune evasion strategies of paramyxoviruses

Immune evasion plays a crucial role in the pathogenicity of paramyxoviruses, presenting significant challenges in the development of effective vaccines and therapeutics. Paramyxoviruses employ various strategies to subvert both innate and adaptive immune responses, including modulation of host-cell interactions and immune suppression. The following key mechanisms of immune evasion are used by paramyxoviruses, with particular focus on their impact on both innate and adaptive immunity.

4.1 Evasion of innate immunity

Innate immunity is the body's first line of defense against viral infections. This defense system involves the activation of pattern recognition receptors (PRRs) like Toll-like receptors (TLRs) and RIG-I-like receptors (RLRs), which detect viral RNA and trigger the production of type I interferons (IFNs) and pro-inflammatory cytokines. Despite this, paramyxoviruses have evolved several mechanisms to circumvent these immune responses.

4.1.1 Suppression of antiviral pathways

C Protein and accessory proteins interfere with the activation of other innate immune sensors, such as RIG-I and TLRs, which are responsible for detecting viral RNA and initiating antiviral signaling pathways [56, 57].

4.1.2 Interferon (IFN) antagonism

The inhibition of the host's interferon response is a central immune evasion strategy of paramyxoviruses. Viral proteins produced by paramyxoviruses inhibit the activity of interferons and downstream antiviral pathways, preventing the effective initiation of the immune response.

The V protein plays a crucial role in antagonizing IFN production. It inhibits Melanoma Differentiation-Associated protein 5 (MDA5), a cytoplasmic RNA sensor, preventing the activation of type I IFN production. Additionally, the V protein blocks the phosphorylation and activation of interferon regulatory factors (IRFs), which prevents the transcription of interferon-stimulated genes (ISGs) [58–60].

Signal transducer and activator of transcription 2 (STAT2) inhibition: The V protein also targets and degrades STAT2, a key component of the IFN response. In CDV, STAT2 plays a more significant role in IFN responses than STAT1, and its inhibition by the V protein is essential for the virus's ability to evade immune detection [61–63]. By disrupting the STAT2-IRF complex, the virus effectively disables the host's antiviral response.

4.1.3 Additional mechanisms of immune evasion

Complement system evasion: Some paramyxoviruses produce proteins that inhibit complement activation, preventing immune-mediated lysis of infected cells and enhancing viral persistence [64].

Immunosuppressive cytokine production: Certain paramyxoviruses induce the production of immunosuppressive cytokines like interleukin-10 (IL-10), which inhibit immune activation and promote immune tolerance, further aiding in viral persistence [65].

4.2 Modulation of adaptive immunity

4.2.1 Lymphocyte interference

Paramyxoviruses target lymphocytes, such as T cells and dendritic cells, disrupting the adaptive immune response. Viruses like CDV and MV use viral F and H proteins to mediate fusion with host cells, targeting immune cells *via* specific receptors, such as SLAM (CD150) and CD46 found on T cells, B cells, dendritic cells, and macrophages [21, 66]. By infecting myeloid dendritic cells (BDCA-1+ and BDCA-3+), paramyxoviruses impair the ability of these cells to present viral antigens and activate T cells, weakening the adaptive immune response [67]. This leads to T cell suppression, making the host more vulnerable to secondary infections, as seen in MV infections. Infecting T cells leads to decreased cytokine production and activation [21, 66, 68]. This further contributes to immune suppression, promoting viral persistence and increasing susceptibility to secondary infections, as observed in MV infections, where a compromised immune system predisposes individuals to other infections.

4.2.2 Antibody escape mechanisms

Paramyxoviruses have developed strategies to evade neutralizing antibodies, a key part of the adaptive immune response:

Antigenic variation: The viral F (fusion) and H (hemagglutinin) glycoproteins undergo structural changes that reduce the binding affinity of neutralizing antibodies, allowing the virus to evade antibody-mediated neutralization [69]. This variation supports viral persistence and reinfection.

Fusion/Entry complex adaptation: The F protein undergoes conformational changes to facilitate fusion with host cells and reduce the binding affinity of neutralizing antibodies, helping the virus continue to spread while evading immune detection [69].

Antibody-mediated enhancement (ADE): Antibody-mediated enhancement (ADE) in paramyxoviruses occurs when non-neutralizing antibodies facilitate viral entry into immune cells, such as macrophages, by binding to Fc receptors. This process enhances viral infection, leading to increased replication and potentially more severe disease. While ADE has been observed in some paramyxoviruses, such as respiratory syncytial virus (RSV), it is less commonly seen in others like measles [70–72]. In these cases, suboptimal antibody responses or prior exposure can increase the risk of ADE. Despite this, paramyxoviruses generally elicit strong immune responses, and the risk of ADE is relatively low, particularly with effective vaccination. Nonetheless, understanding ADE in paramyxoviruses remains important, especially in cases of incomplete immunity or suboptimal vaccine responses [70].

In conclusion, paramyxoviruses employ a wide array of sophisticated immune evasion strategies to overcome both innate and adaptive immune defenses. These strategies include the inhibition of interferon production, suppression of antiviral pathways, disruption of lymphocyte function, and evasion of antibody-mediated neutralization. By targeting key immune mechanisms, such as interferon signaling and dendritic cell function, paramyxoviruses can persist in the host and evade immune surveillance. Although antibody-dependent enhancement (ADE) is relatively rare, it remains an important consideration, particularly in cases of incomplete immunity or suboptimal vaccination. A deeper understanding of these immune evasion tactics is crucial for the development of more effective vaccines and antiviral treatments to combat paramyxoviral infections.

5. Vaccines

Vaccination strategies have played a pivotal role in mitigating the impact of many of these pathogens, although challenges remain in developing vaccines that are both universally applicable and capable of addressing emerging viral variants.

5.1 Types of paramyxovirus vaccines

Vaccines for paramyxoviruses can be broadly categorized into several types based on their composition and mode of action. The categories of paramyxovirus vaccination are addressed as follows. Each vaccine type presents distinct advantages and drawbacks, depending on the viral target, the environmental conditions of vaccine deployment, and the desired immune response.

5.1.1 Inactivated vaccines

Inactivated vaccines consist of viruses that have been chemically or physically inactivated, rendering them noninfectious while retaining their immunogenic properties. These vaccines typically require the inclusion of adjuvants to enhance immune responses. Although inactivated vaccines are general considered safe, they tend to induce shorter-duration immunity compared to live-attenuated vaccines and often necessitate booster doses. For example, the inactivated PPRV vaccines offer effective control of outbreaks but are associated with limited long-term immunity [73]. Likewise, the NDV (B1 strain) is also widely used in regions where live vaccines may pose a higher risk. These inactivated vaccines are safe but induce weaker immune responses compared to their live-attenuated counterparts **Table 1** [74–76]. Advantages and disadvantages of different paramyxovirus vaccine types. Limitations: Short-lived immunity, reliance on adjuvants, lack of differentiating infected from vaccinated animals (DIVA) capability.

5.1.2 Live-attenuated vaccines

Live-attenuated vaccines utilize viruses that have been weakened through serial passage or genetic modification to reduce pathogenicity. These vaccines generally induce robust immune responses, including both humoral and cellular immunity, and

Vaccine type	Advantages	Disadvantages
Inactivated Vaccines	• Low risk of reversion to virulence • Safe for immunocompromised populations • Stable in storage	• Immunity is short-lived • Requires adjuvants • No DIVA capability • Boosters needed
Live-Attenuated Vaccines	• Provides long-lasting immunity • Induces strong humoral and cellular immune responses • Mimics natural infection	• Risk of reversion to virulence • Requires cold storage • No DIVA capability • Risk in immunocompromised individuals
Thermostable Vaccines	• Stable at varying temperatures • Suitable for areas with limited refrigeration • Ideal for low-resource settings	• Efficacy may be affected by poor storage • Still needs temperature control
Recombinant Vaccines	• Safer than live-attenuated vaccines • DIVA capability • Lower risk of adverse reactions • Flexible production	• Reduced efficacy in some cases • Some are still under development for certain pathogens
Virus-Like Particles (VLPs)	• Noninfectious • Mimics virus structure • Safe and does not require biocontainment • Strong immune response like a natural infection	• Still in development • Immunogenicity can vary • Expensive production
mRNA Vaccines	• Rapid development • No infection risk from the vaccine • Can adapt to emerging pathogens • Broad applicability across viruses	• Requires ultra • Cold storage • Limited real-world experience • New technology
Chimeric Vaccines	• Immunity to multiple viruses • Allows DIVA • Can address co-infections	• Potentially short-lived immunity • Requires further optimization and research
Subunit Vaccines	• Safe (no live virus) • Lower risk of adverse reactions • Targets specific viral proteins	• Requires adjuvants • May not offer long-lasting immunity • Requires booster doses

Table 1.
Advantages and disadvantages of different paramyxovirus vaccine types.

often provide long-lasting protection. However, concerns regarding the reversion of the virus to a virulent form and the requirement for cold storage pose challenges.

For example, PPRV (Live-attenuated) vaccines offer long-lasting immunity but are thermolabile and require stringent cold chain management [73]. Similarly, the NDV (La Sota strain) is a well-established vaccine in poultry, which induces strong immune responses but carries the risk of virus reversion to virulence [75]. The CDV (Rockborn and Schneider strains) were commonly used to prevent distemper in canines these vaccines provide effective protection but may present risks in certain immunocompromised populations [77].

Advantages: Durable immunity, mimics natural infection, robust immune response.

Limitations: Risk of reversion to virulence, storage requirements, no DIVA capability.

5.1.3 Thermostable vaccines

Thermostable vaccines are designed to maintain their efficacy under varying temperature conditions, making them suitable for use in regions with limited access to refrigeration. These vaccines are particularly important for the distribution of vaccines in remote areas or low-resource settings.

For example, I-2 vaccine for NDV, is a thermostable live-attenuated vaccine that is resistant to temperature fluctuations, ensuring its viability during transport and storage in areas with inadequate cold chain infrastructure [74, 75].

Advantages: Stability under fluctuating temperatures, ideal for regions with limited refrigeration.

Limitations: Efficacy may vary depending on environmental conditions, storage still requires temperature control.

5.1.4 Recombinant vaccines

Recombinant vaccines involve the genetic engineering of viral antigens into vectors, typically attenuated viruses, to stimulate an immune response without the risks associated with live viral infections. These vaccines can enable DIVA, which is crucial for distinguishing between infected and vaccinated animals.

For example, the PPRV (Recombinant Vaccines using MVA, Baculovirus) [73], NDV (Fowlpox virus-based recombinant vaccines) [75], and CDV (Recombinant vaccines combining live and inactivated strains) [77].

Advantages: Safer than live-attenuated vaccines, DIVA capability, reduced risk of adverse reactions.

Limitations: Reduced efficacy in certain cases, ongoing development for specific pathogens.

5.1.5 Virus-like particles (VLPs)

Virus-like particles are molecular structures that mimic the architecture of a virus but lack viral genomic material, rendering them noninfectious. VLP vaccines (e.g., the NDV VLPs [75] and PPRV VLPs [73]) have the potential to elicit strong immune responses similar to natural infection, without the associated risk of live virus transmission.

Advantages: Safe, noninfectious, mimics natural virus structure, no requirement for biocontainment facilities.

Limitations: Still under development, variable immunogenicity.

5.1.6 mRNA vaccines

mRNA vaccines utilize synthetic messenger RNA that encodes viral antigens, which are then expressed in the host cells to stimulate an immune response. This technology allows for rapid vaccine development, as demonstrated by the success of mRNA vaccines against SARS-CoV-2, and is now being explored for various paramyxoviruses (e.g., HRSV Moderna's mRNA-1653) [78] and PIV3 and HMPV mRNA vaccines [78].

Advantages: Rapid development, adaptability to emerging pathogens, and no risk of infection from the vaccine.

Limitations: Limited real-world experience, requires ultra-cold storage, and relatively new technology.

5.1.7 Chimeric vaccines

Chimeric vaccines are genetically engineered to combine components from different viruses to create a hybrid vaccine capable of inducing immunity against multiple pathogens (e.g., the RPV- PPRV Chimeric Vaccine [73]). These vaccines may also facilitate DIVA, offering an advantage in surveillance and control efforts.

Advantages: Immunity to multiple viruses, enables DIVA.

Limitations: Potentially short-lived immunity, requires additional research for optimization.

5.1.8 Subunit vaccines

Subunit vaccines For example, the HeV and NiV (glycoprotein-based subunit vaccines) and RSV (HRSV subunit vaccines) [79, 80] consist of purified viral proteins, typically glycoproteins, which are sufficient to stimulate an immune response without using the whole virus. These vaccines are particularly valuable for pathogens that pose significant safety risks, as they eliminate the need for live viral material.

Advantages: Safe, no live virus, reduced adverse reactions.

Limitations: Requires adjuvants, may not provide long-lasting immunity.

The development of vaccines for paramyxoviruses has made significant strides, with various vaccine platforms now available or under development. While live-attenuated vaccines remain the most widely used due to their efficacy, novel vaccine strategies such as recombinant, mRNA, and virus-like particle-based vaccines show promise in addressing some of the limitations of traditional approaches. The continued advancement of these vaccine technologies is crucial for enhancing global efforts to control paramyxovirus-related diseases, particularly in regions with limited healthcare infrastructure.

5.2 Challenges in vaccine development

The development of vaccines for paramyxoviruses faces several scientific and practical challenges despite notable progress. One significant hurdle is the variability in vaccine efficacy, as the effectiveness of vaccines can differ depending on the circulating viral strains. For instance, the La Sota strain of Newcastle disease virus (NDV) is protective against some strains but not universally effective due to antigenic differences. Additionally, viruses like Nipah (NiV) and Hendra (HeV) pose a high zoonotic risk, requiring vaccines that are effective in both animals and humans to prevent spillover, which is complicated by the variability of immune responses. Another challenge is achieving the right balance in the immune response; over-attenuated vaccines may not stimulate enough immunity, while under-attenuated vaccines can lead to adverse effects, as seen with respiratory syncytial virus (RSV) vaccines, which cause wheezing in infants.

Large-scale production of live-attenuated or inactivated viruses for vaccines remains difficult, especially in low-resource settings, necessitating efficient systems to meet global demand. Maternal antibodies can also interfere with vaccine efficacy in infants, making it crucial to develop vaccines that can overcome this barrier to ensure protection early in life. Furthermore, vaccine hesitancy has contributed to the resurgence of diseases like measles and mumps, highlighting the need for public education and transparent communication. The risk of reversion to virulence in live-attenuated vaccines, such as with NDV, also presents a concern, as outbreaks have occurred due to the vaccine strain reverting. In large-scale vaccination programs, like those for poultry, simultaneous vaccination can lead to interference, reducing the effectiveness of one or both vaccines.

Lastly, ensuring long-lasting immunity without causing excessive inflammation is a challenge, as some paramyxovirus vaccines, such as those for mumps or measles, may lose efficacy over time and require booster doses. Overcoming these challenges in efficacy, safety, production, and zoonotic transmission will require innovative approaches in vaccine design, production, and surveillance to provide broad, effective protection for both humans and animals.

6. Antiviral strategies for paramyxovirus infections

Despite the availability of vaccines for certain paramyxoviruses, antiviral therapy remains an important area of research due to the absence of effective treatments for many paramyxovirus infections. The high morbidity, particularly in immunocompromised individuals or populations lacking vaccination, emphasizes the need for effective antiviral treatments.

The paramyxovirus lifecycle begins when the virus binds to host cell receptors through its attachment.

(H) protein and subsequently fuses with the cell membrane *via* the F protein. Once inside, the viral RNA genome is released, and the virus hijacks the host's cellular machinery for replication. The newly formed viral proteins and RNA genomes are then packaged into new virions, which exit the host cell and spread the infection to other cells. This process is tightly regulated and presents several potential targets for antiviral intervention. The viral fusion process, replication machinery, and interactions with host immune responses are all critical components in the viral lifecycle that can be disrupted by antiviral therapies.

6.1 Antiviral approaches targeting the fusion (F) protein

The viral fusion (F) protein is a key player in paramyxovirus entry and is a major target for antiviral development. This protein undergoes conformational changes that allow the virus to fuse with the host cell membrane, facilitating infection. Inhibiting this process prevents viral entry and replication.

a. *Fusion-inhibitory peptides*: Fusion-inhibitory peptides are designed to bind to the F protein and block the conformational changes required for viral fusion. These peptides are effective in preventing viral entry into host cells [81]. Recent studies have shown that broad-spectrum fusion inhibitors targeting the paramyxovirus F protein can be effective against multiple paramyxovirus strains, including RSV, NDV, and measles [81, 82].

b. *Small-molecule inhibitors*: Small-molecule inhibitors targeting the F protein have emerged as an important therapeutic approach. These molecules are typically designed to interfere with the interaction between the viral F protein and the host cell membrane, preventing the fusion process. For example, inhibitors like palivizumab (used for RSV) and other experimental small molecules have shown promise in blocking viral fusion, thereby preventing infection [83–85].

6.2 Antiviral strategies targeting viral replication

After fusion and release of the viral genome, paramyxoviruses replicate their RNA genome inside the host cell. Inhibition of viral RNA polymerase or other enzymes involved in replication is another therapeutic strategy.

a. *RNA polymerase or replication complex inhibitors*: The polymerase complex, consisting of the L and P proteins, is essential for transcription and replication of viral RNA, making it a key target for antiviral therapies. Nucleoside analogs like favipiravir and ribavirin work by terminating RNA chains [86, 87], while non-nucleoside inhibitors disrupt the paramyxovirus RNA polymerase complex [88]. However, challenges such as resistance and host toxicity remain.

   Recent research has identified new antiviral agents targeting other viral proteins, such as the F and M proteins, which are crucial for viral fusion and assembly. For example, Nitazoxanide has shown broad-spectrum activity by interfering with the folding of these proteins [89].

b. *Host-targeted antiviral agents*: Another strategy is to target host cell proteins that paramyxoviruses rely on for replication. Host-targeted antiviral agents are designed to inhibit the activity of cellular factors that viruses manipulate to replicate their RNA genomes. Recent studies suggest that the host protein viperin, an enzyme involved in antiviral defense, can be targeted to inhibit paramyxovirus replication [90, 91].

6.3 Immune modulation and host immune response

One of the hallmarks of paramyxovirus infection is the ability to evade the host's immune response, particularly the innate immune system. Paramyxoviruses encode a variety of proteins that inhibit the host's interferon response and other immune defenses.

a. *Inhibition of immune evasion proteins*: The V protein of paramyxoviruses, such as measles virus (MV) and RSV, plays a critical role in immune evasion by blocking interferon production and disrupting the host's antiviral immune response [92]. Therapeutic strategies targeting these viral immune modulators, such as small molecules or monoclonal antibodies, have the potential to restore the immune system's ability to fight off the infection.

b. *Cytokine modulation*: Certain antiviral strategies focus on modulating the immune response to enhance host defenses [93]. For example, the use of immune adjuvants or cytokine therapies can boost the production of interferons and other cytokines, helping to restore the body's innate immune response against paramyxoviruses.

6.4 Challenges and future directions

Despite significant advances in antiviral drug development, there are several challenges in the treatment of paramyxovirus infections. One of the major challenges is the rapid mutation of viruses, which can lead to drug resistance. Another obstacle is the difficulty in delivering antiviral drugs effectively, particularly for respiratory infections like RSV, where delivery to the site of infection is crucial.

The development of broad-spectrum antiviral agents that target conserved viral mechanisms, such as the F protein, is a key focus of future research. Additionally, enhancing vaccine strategies and combining antiviral therapy with immunotherapies to modulate the host immune response may provide more effective treatments for paramyxovirus infections in the future. Ultimately, a multi-pronged approach involving antiviral drugs, vaccines, and immune therapies will be essential in combating the global threat posed by paramyxoviruses.

7. Conclusions

In conclusion, morbilliviruses, members of the Paramyxoviridae family, exhibit a complex interplay with host immune systems that facilitates their persistence and pathogenesis. Viral replication involves several key steps, including attachment to host cells *via* receptor interactions, fusion with the host cell membrane, and subsequent RNA replication and transcription within the cytoplasm. These processes culminate in virion assembly and release. The ability of morbilliviruses to evade immune responses, particularly through the suppression of type I interferon signaling and manipulation of immune cell function, complicates both therapeutic interventions and vaccine development. Despite advances in the development of vaccines and antiviral strategies, challenges such as immune evasion mechanisms, viral strain variability, and accessibility to treatments in resource-limited settings remain. Continued research into the molecular mechanisms underlying morbillivirus replication, immune modulation, and host-virus interactions is essential for the design of more effective vaccines and antiviral therapies. A multi-pronged approach, incorporating improved vaccines, antiviral agents, and immune modulatory treatments, is crucial for controlling morbillivirus infections and mitigating their impact on both human and veterinary populations.

Author details

Ashok Kumar[1], Ram Kumar[2], Anil Gattani[3*] and Sanju Mandal[4]

1 Animal Disease Research Centre, Guru Angad Dev Veterinary and Animal Sciences University, Ludhiana, Punjab, India

2 Department of Veterinary Microbiology, Rajasthan University of Veterinary and Animal Sciences, Bikaner, Rajasthan, India

3 Department of Veterinary Physiology and Biochemistry, Nanaji Deshmukh Veterinary Science University, Jabalpur, India

4 Department of Veterinary Physiology and Biochemistry, CoVSc and AH, The Nanaji Deshmukh Veterinary Science University, Jabalpur, India

*Address all correspondence to: gattanianil@gmail.com

References

[1] Parija SC. Paramyxoviruses. In: Textbook of Microbiology and Immunology. Singapore: Springer Nature Singapore; 2023. pp. 811-824. DOI: 10.1007/978-981-19-3315-8_57

[2] Liu D. Classification of medically important viruses. In: Molecular Medical Microbiology. Academic Press; 2024. pp. 2061-2072. DOI: 10.1016/B978-0-12-818619-0.00161-1

[3] Fermin G. Virion structure, genome organization, and taxonomy of viruses. Viruses. 2018;**17**:17-54. DOI: 10.1016/B978-0-12-811257-1.00002-4

[4] De Vries RD, Duprex WP, De Swart RL. Morbillivirus infections: An introduction. Viruses. 2015;7(2):699-706. DOI: 10.3390/v7020699

[5] Dicker K, Järvelin AI, Garcia-Moreno M, Castello A. The importance of virion-incorporated cellular RNA-binding proteins in viral particle assembly and infectivity. In: Seminars in Cell and Developmental Biology. Vol. 111. Academic Press; 2021. pp. 108-118. DOI: 10.1016/j.semcdb.2020.08.002

[6] Dolnik O, Gerresheim GK, Biedenkopf N. New perspectives on the biogenesis of viral inclusion bodies in negative-sense RNA virus infections. Cells. 2021;**10**(6):1460. DOI: 10.3390/cells10061460

[7] Barrett T, Banyard AC, Diallo A. Molecular biology of the morbilliviruses. In: Rinderpest and peste des petits Ruminants. Academic Press; 2006. pp. 31-IV. DOI: 10.1016/B978-012088385-1/50033-2

[8] Kumar N, Maherchandani S, Kashyap SK, Singh SV, Sharma S, Chaubey KK, et al. Peste des petits ruminants virus infection of small ruminants: A comprehensive review. Viruses. 2014;**6**(6):2287-2327. DOI: 10.3390/v6062287

[9] Manjunath S, Kumar GR, Mishra BP, Mishra B, Sahoo AP, Joshi CG, et al. Genomic analysis of host–Peste des petits ruminants vaccine viral transcriptome uncovers transcription factors modulating immune regulatory pathways. Veterinary Research. 2015;**46**:1-15. DOI: 10.1186/s13567-015-0153-8

[10] Sourimant J, Plemper RK. Organization, function, and therapeutic targeting of the morbillivirus RNA-dependent RNA polymerase complex. Viruses. 2016;**8**(9):251. DOI: 10.3390/v8090251

[11] Vanmechelen B. Virus Discovery in Small Mammals: A Closer Look at the Families Arteriviridae and Paramyxoviridae. Faculty of Veterinary Medicine, Ghent University; 2022

[12] Pfaller CK, Cattaneo R, Schnell MJ. Reverse genetics of Mononegavirales: How they work, new vaccines, and new cancer therapeutics. Virology. 2015;**479**:331-344. DOI: 10.1016/j.virol.2015.01.029

[13] Yadav AK, Rajak KK, Bhatt M, Kumar A, Chakravarti S, Sankar M, et al. Comparative sequence analysis of morbillivirus receptors and its implication in host range expansion. Canadian Journal of Microbiology. 2019;**65**(11):783-794. DOI: 10.1139/cjm-2019-0008

[14] Gaur SK, Jain J, Chaudhary Y, Kaul R. Insights into the mechanism of Morbillivirus induced immune

suppression. Virology. 2024;**110212**:14-110212. DOI: 10.1016/j.virol.2024.110212

[15] Tatsuo H, Yanagi Y. The morbillivirus receptor SLAM (CD150). Microbiology and Immunology. 2002;**46**(3):135-142. DOI: 10.1111/j.1348-0421.2002.tb02678.x

[16] Von Messling V, Svitek N, Cattaneo R. Receptor (SLAM [CD150]) recognition and the V protein sustain swift lymphocyte-based invasion of mucosal tissue and lymphatic organs by a morbillivirus. Journal of Virology. 2006;**80**(12):6084-6092. DOI: 10.1128/jvi.00357-06

[17] Aversa G, Chang CC, Carballido JM, Cocks BG, de Vries JE. Engagement of the signaling lymphocytic activation molecule (SLAM) on activated T cells results in IL-2-independent, cyclosporin A-sensitive T cell proliferation and IFN-gamma production. Journal of Immunology (Baltimore, Md.: 1950). 1997;**158**(9):4036-4044

[18] Wu N, Veillette A. SLAM family receptors in normal immunity and immune pathologies. Current Opinion in Immunology. 2016;**38**:45-51. DOI: 10.1016/j.coi.2015.11.003

[19] Massé N, Ainouze M, Néel B, Wild TF, Buckland R, Langedijk JP. Measles virus (MV) hemagglutinin: Evidence that attachment sites for MV receptors SLAM and CD46 overlap on the globular head. Journal of Virology. 2004;**78**(17):9051-9063. DOI: 10.1128/JVI.78.17.9051-9063.2004

[20] Sato H, Yoneda M, Honda T, Kai C. Morbillivirus receptors and tropism: Multiple pathways for infection. Frontiers in Microbiology. 2012;**3**:75. DOI: 10.3389/fmicb.2012.00075

[21] Tatsuo H, Ono N, Yanagi Y. Morbilliviruses use signaling lymphocyte activation molecules (CD150) as cellular receptors. Journal of Virology. 2001;**75**(13):5842-5850. DOI: 10.1128/JVI.75.13.5842-5850.2001

[22] Adombi CM, Lelenta M, Lamien CE, Shamaki D, Koffi YM, Traoré A, et al. Monkey CV1 cell line expressing the sheep–goat SLAM protein: A highly sensitive cell line for the isolation of peste des petits ruminants virus from pathological specimens. Journal of Virological Methods. 2011;**173**(2):306-313. DOI: 10.1016/j.jviromet.2011.02.024

[23] Yanagi Y, Takeda M, Ohno S. Measles virus: Cellular receptors, tropism and pathogenesis. Journal of General Virus. 2006;**87**(10):2767-2779. DOI: 10.1099/vir.0.82221-0

[24] Leonard VH, Sinn PL, Hodge G, Miest T, Devaux P, Oezguen N, et al. Measles virus blind to its epithelial cell receptor remains virulent in rhesus monkeys but cannot cross the airway epithelium and is not shed. The Journal of Clinical Investigation. 2008;**118**(7):2448-2458. DOI: 10.1172/JCI35454

[25] Tahara M, Ito Y, Brindley MA, Ma X, He J, Xu S, et al. Functional and structural characterization of neutralizing epitopes of measles virus hemagglutinin protein. Journal of Virology. 2013;**87**(1):666-675. DOI: 10.1128/JVI.02033-12

[26] Pfeffermann K, Doerr M, Zirkel F, von Messling V. Morbillivirus pathogenesis and virus–host interactions. Advances in Virus Research. 2018;**100**:75-98. DOI: 10.1016/bs.aivir.2017.12.003

[27] Noyce RS, Richardson CD. Nectin 4 is the epithelial cell receptor for measles virus. Trends in Microbiology. 2012;**20**(9):429-439. DOI: 10.1016/j.tim.2012.05.006

[28] Mühlebach MD, Mateo M, Sinn PL, Prüfer S, Uhlig KM, Leonard VH, et al. Adherens junction protein nectin-4 is the epithelial receptor for measles virus. Nature. 2011;**480**(7378):530-533. DOI: 10.1038/nature10639

[29] Fujita K, Miura R, Yoneda M, Shimizu F, Sato H, Muto Y, et al. Host range and receptor utilization of canine distemper virus analyzed by recombinant viruses: Involvement of heparin-like molecule in CDV infection. Virology. 2007;**359**(2):324-335. DOI: 10.1016/j.virol.2006.09.018

[30] Yanagi Y, Ono N, Tatsuo H, Hashimoto K, Minagawa H. Measles virus receptor SLAM (CD150). Virology. 2002;**299**(2):155-161. DOI: 10.1006/viro.2002.1471

[31] Abdullah N, Kelly JT, Graham SC, Birch J, Gonçalves-Carneiro D, Mitchell T, et al. Structure-guided identification of a nonhuman morbillivirus with zoonotic potential. Journal of Virology. 2018;**92**(23):10-1128. DOI: 10.1128/JVI.01248-18

[32] Ader-Ebert N, Khosravi M, Herren M, Avila M, Alves L, Bringolf F, et al. Sequential conformational changes in the morbillivirus attachment protein initiate the membrane fusion process. PLoS Pathogens. 2015;**11**(5):e1004880. DOI: 10.1371/journal.ppat.1004880

[33] Navaratnarajah CK, Generous AR, Yousaf I, Cattaneo R. Receptor-mediated cell entry of paramyxoviruses: Mechanisms, and consequences for tropism and pathogenesis. The Journal of Biological Chemistry. 2020 Feb 28;**295**(9):2771-2786. Epub 2020 Jan 16. DOI: 10.1074/jbc.REV119.009961

[34] Kim CH, Kim CH. Viral protein interaction with host cells GSLs. Glycosphingolipids Signaling. 2020:53-92. DOI: 10.1007/978-981-15-5807-8_4

[35] Zinzula L, Beck F, Klumpe S, Bohn S, Pfeifer G, Bollschweiler D, et al. Cryo-EM structure of the cetacean morbillivirus nucleoprotein-RNA complex. Journal of Structural Biology. 2021;**213**(3):107750. DOI: 10.1016/j.jsb.2021.107750

[36] Munir M, Zohari S, Berg M, Munir M, Zohari S, Berg M. Genome organization of peste des petits ruminants virus. In: Molecular Biology and Pathogenesis of Peste Des Petits Ruminants Virus. 2013. pp. 1-22. DOI: 10.1007/978-3-642-31451-3_1

[37] Kozak M. Selection of initiation sites by eucaryotic ribosomes: Effect of inserting AUG triplets upstream from the coding sequence for preproinsulin. Nucleic Acids Research. 1984;**12**(9):3873-3893. DOI: 10.1093/nar/12.9.3873

[38] Schneider-Schaulies J. Cellular receptors for viruses: Links to tropism and pathogenesis. Journal of General Virology. 2000;**81**(6):1413-1429. DOI: 10.1099/0022-1317-81-6-1413

[39] Wertz GW, Perepelitsa VP, Ball LA. Gene rearrangement attenuates expression and lethality of a nonsegmented negative strand RNA virus. Proceedings of the National Academy of Sciences. 1998;**95**(7):3501-3506. DOI: 10.1073/pnas.95.7.3501

[40] Kolakofsky D, Le Mercier P, Iseni F, Garcin D. Viral RNA polymerase scanning and the gymnastics of Sendai virus RNA synthesis. Virology. 2004;**318**(2):463-473. DOI: 10.1016/j.virol.2003.10.031

[41] Maclachlan NJ, Dubovi EJ, editors. Fenner's Veterinary Virology. Academic Press; 2010

[42] Vincent S, Gerlier D, Manié SN. Measles virus assembly within membrane rafts. Journal of Virology. 2000;**74**(21):9911-9915. DOI: 10.1128/jvi.74.21.9911-9915.2000

[43] Laliberte JP, McGinnes LW, Morrison TG. Incorporation of functional HN-F glycoprotein-containing complexes into Newcastle disease virus is dependent on cholesterol and membrane lipid raft integrity. Journal of Virology. 2007;**81**(19):10636-10648. DOI: 10.1128/JVI.01119-07

[44] Pohl C, Duprex WP, Krohne G, Rima BK, Schneider-Schaulies S. Measles virus M and F proteins associate with detergent-resistant membrane fractions and promote formation of virus-like particles. Journal of General Virology. 2007;**88**(4):1243-1250. DOI: 10.1099/vir.0.82578-0

[45] El Najjar F, Schmitt AP, Dutch RE. Paramyxovirus glycoprotein incorporation, assembly and budding: A three way dance for infectious particle production. Viruses. 2014;**6**(8):3019-3054. DOI: 10.3390/v608301

[46] Rossman JS, Lamb RA. Viral membrane scission. Annual Review of Cell and Developmental Biology. 2013;**29**(1):551-569. DOI: 10.1146/annurev-cellbio-101011-155838

[47] Harrison MS, Sakaguchi T, Schmitt AP. Paramyxovirus assembly and budding: Building particles that transmit infections. The International Journal of Biochemistry and Cell Biology. 2010;**42**(9):1416-1429. DOI: 10.1016/j.biocel.2010.04.005

[48] Takimoto T, Portner A. Molecular mechanism of paramyxovirus budding. Virus Research. 2004;**106**(2):133-145

[49] Duan Z, Hu Z, Zhu J, Xu H, Chen J, Liu H, et al. Mutations in the FPIV motif of Newcastle disease virus matrix protein attenuate virus replication and reduce virus budding. Archives of Virology. 2014;**159**:1813-1819. DOI: 10.1007/s00705-014-1998-2

[50] Salditt A, Koethe S, Pohl C, Harms H, Kolesnikova L, Becker S, et al. Measles virus M protein-driven particle production does not involve the endosomal sorting complex required for transport (ESCRT) system. Journal of General Virology. 2010;**91**(6):1464-1472. DOI: 10.1099/vir.0.018523-0

[51] Fouillot-Coriou N, Roux L. Structure–function analysis of the Sendai virus F and HN cytoplasmic domain: Different role for the two proteins in the production of virus particle. Virology. 2000;**270**(2):464-475. DOI: 10.1006/viro.2000.0291

[52] Essaidi-Laziosi M, Shevtsova A, Gerlier D, Roux L. Mutation of the TYTLE motif in the cytoplasmic tail of the Sendai virus fusion protein deeply affects viral assembly and particle production. PLoS One. 2013;**8**(12):e78074. DOI: 10.1371/journal.pone.0078074

[53] Liljeroos L, Krzyzaniak MA, Helenius A, Butcher SJ. Architecture of respiratory syncytial virus revealed by electron cryotomography. Proceedings of the National Academy of Sciences. 2013;**110**(27):11133-11138. DOI: 10.1073/pnas.1309070110

[54] Gonçalves Carneiro VD. Molecular Mechanisms of Measles Virus Entry and Exit (Doctoral Dissertation, University of Birmingham). 2017. Available from: http://etheses.bham.ac.uk/id/eprint/7514

[55] Naim HY, Ehler E, Billeter MA. Measles virus matrix protein specifies apical virus release and glycoprotein

sorting in epithelial cells. The EMBO Journal. 2000;**19**(14):3576-3585. DOI: 10.1093/emboj/19.14.3576

[56] Parks GD, Alexander-Miller MA. Paramyxovirus activation and inhibition of innate immune responses. Journal of Molecular Biology. 2013;**425**(24):4872-4892. DOI: 10.1016/j.jmb.2013.09.015

[57] Siering O, Cattaneo R, Pfaller CK. C proteins: Controllers of orderly paramyxovirus replication and of the innate immune response. Viruses. 2022;**14**(1):137. DOI: 10.3390/v14010137

[58] Childs K, Andrejeva J, Randall RE, Goodbourn S. Mechanism of mda-5 inhibition by paramyxovirus V proteins. Journal of Virology. 2009;**83**(3):1465-1473. DOI: 10.1128/JVI.01768-08

[59] Devasthanam AS. Mechanisms underlying the inhibition of interferon signaling by viruses. Virulence. 2014;**5**(2):270-277. DOI: 10.4161/viru.27902

[60] Ramachandran A, Horvath CM. Dissociation of paramyxovirus interferon evasion activities: Universal and virus-specific requirements for conserved V protein amino acids in MDA5 interference. Journal of Virology. 2010;**84**(21):11152-11163. DOI: 10.1128/JVI.01375-10

[61] Andrejeva J, Young D, Goodbourn S, Randall RE. Degradation of STAT1 and STAT2 by the V proteins of simian virus 5 and human parainfluenza virus type 2, respectively: Consequences for virus replication in the presence of alpha/beta and gamma interferons. Journal of Virology. 2002;**76**(5):2159-2167. DOI: 10.1128/jvi.76.5.2159-2167.2002

[62] Ma X, Yang X, Nian X, Zhang Z, Dou Y, Zhang X, et al. Identification of amino-acid residues in the V protein of peste des petits ruminants essential for interference and suppression of STAT-mediated interferon signaling. Virology. 2015;**483**:54-63. DOI: 10.1016/j.virol.2015.03.039

[63] Röthlisberger A, Wiener D, Schweizer M, Peterhans E, Zurbriggen A, Plattet P. Two domains of the V protein of virulent canine distemper virus selectively inhibit STAT1 and STAT2 nuclear import. Journal of Virology. 2010;**84**(13):6328-6343. DOI: 10.1128/JVI.01878-09

[64] Agrawal P, Nawadkar R, Ojha H, Kumar J, Sahu A. Complement evasion strategies of viruses: An overview. Frontiers in Microbiology. 2017;**8**:1117. DOI: 10.3389/fmicb.2017.01117

[65] Ng SSM, Li A, Pavlakis GN, Ozato K, Kino T. Viral infection increases glucocorticoid-induced interleukin-10 production through ERK-mediated phosphorylation of the glucocorticoid receptor in dendritic cells: Potential clinical implications. PLoS One. 2013;**8**(5):e63587. DOI: 10.1371/journal.pone.0063587

[66] Schneider-Schaulies J, Schneider-Schaulies S. Receptor interactions, tropism, and mechanisms involved in morbillivirus-induced immunomodulation. Advances in Virus Research. 2008;**71**:173-205. DOI: 10.1016/S0065-3527(08)00004-3

[67] Gupta MR, Kolli D, Molteni C, Casola A, Garofalo RP. Paramyxovirus infection regulates T cell responses by BDCA-1+ and BDCA-3+ myeloid dendritic cells. PLoS One. 2014;**9**(6):e99227. DOI: 10.1371/journal.pone.0099227

[68] Rijks JM, Osterhaus A, Kuiken T, Frölich K. Morbillivirus Infections. Wiley Online Library; 2012. p. 99. DOI: 10.1002/9781118342442

[69] Marcink TC, Zipursky G, Sobolik EB, Golub K, Herman E, Stearns K, et al. How a paramyxovirus fusion/entry complex adapts to escape a neutralizing antibody. Nature Communications. 2024;**15**(1):8831. DOI: 10.1038/s41467-024-53082-y

[70] Banoun H. Measles and antibody-dependent enhancement (ADE): History and mechanisms. In: Exploratory Research and Hypothesis in Medicine. 2022. pp. 000-000. DOI: 10.14218/ERHM.2022.00018

[71] Kulkarni R. Antibody-dependent enhancement of viral infections. In: Dynamics of Immune Activation in Viral Diseases. 2020. pp. 9-41. DOI: 10.1007/978-981-15-1045-8_2

[72] Porterfield JS. Antibody-dependent enhancement of viral infectivity. Advances in Virus Research. 1986;**31**:335-355. DOI: 10.1016/s0065-3527(08)60268-7

[73] Kumar N, Barua S, Riyesh T, Tripathi BN. Advances in peste des petits ruminants vaccines. Veterinary Microbiology. 2017;**206**:91-101. DOI: 10.1016/j.vetmic.2017.01.010

[74] Bala N. Studies on Thermostable Newcastle Disease Virus Induced Cytokine Expression in Chicken Embryo Fibroblastt. Hisar, India: University of Veterinary and Animal Sciences; 2023

[75] Dimitrov KM, Afonso CL, Yu Q, Miller PJ. Newcastle disease vaccines—A solved problem or a continuous challenge? Veterinary Microbiology. 2017;**206**:126-136. DOI: 10.1016/j.vetmic.2016.12.019

[76] Fulber JP, Kamen AA. Development and scalable production of Newcastle disease virus-vectored vaccines for human and veterinary use. Viruses. 2022;**14**(5):975. DOI: 10.3390/v14050975

[77] Martella V, Blixenkrone-Møller M, Elia G, Lucente MS, Cirone F, Decaro N, et al. Lights and shades on an historical vaccine canine distemper virus, the Rockborn strain. Vaccine. 2011;**29**(6):1222-1227. DOI: 10.1016/j.vaccine.2010.12.001

[78] August A, Shaw CA, Lee H, Knightly C, Kalidindia S, Chu L, et al. Safety and immunogenicity of an mRNA-based human metapneumovirus and parainfluenza virus type 3 combined vaccine in healthy adults. Paper Presented at the Open Forum Infectious Diseases. 2022;**7**(9):ofac206. DOI: 10.1093/ofid/ofac206

[79] Hurwitz JL. Respiratory syncytial virus vaccine development. Expert Review of Vaccines. 2011;**10**(10):1415-1433. DOI: 10.1586/erv.11.120

[80] McEachern JA, Bingham J, Crameri G, Green DJ, Hancock TJ, Middleton D, et al. A recombinant subunit vaccine formulation protects against lethal Nipah virus challenge in cats. Vaccine. 2008;**26**(31):3842-3852. DOI: 10.1016/j.vaccine.2008.05.016

[81] Düzgüneş N, Fernandez-Fuentes N, Konopka K. Inhibition of viral membrane fusion by peptides and approaches to peptide design. Pathogens. 2021;**10**(12):1599. DOI: 10.3390/pathogens10121599

[82] Monteiro A, Yu KO, Hicar MD. Peptide-based fusion inhibitors for preventing the six-helix bundle formation of class I fusion proteins: HIV and beyond. Current HIV Research. 2021;**19**(6):465-475. DOI: 10.2174/1570162X19666210908115231

[83] Battles MB, Langedijk JP, Furmanova-Hollenstein P, Chaiwatpongsakorn S, Costello HM, Kwanten L, et al. Molecular mechanism

of respiratory syncytial virus fusion inhibitors. Nature Chemical Biology. 2016;**12**(2):87-93. DOI: 10.1038/nchembio.1982

[84] Elawar F, Oraby AK, Kieser Q, Jensen LD, Culp T, West FG, et al. Pharmacological targets and emerging treatments for respiratory syncytial virus bronchiolitis. Pharmacology and Therapeutics. 2021;**220**:107712. DOI: 10.1016/j.pharmthera.2020.107712

[85] Felicetti T, Sarnari C, Gaito R, Tabarrini O, Manfroni G. Recent progress toward the discovery of small molecules as novel anti-respiratory syncytial virus agents. Journal of Medicinal Chemistry. 2024;**67**(14):11543-11579. DOI: 10.1021/acs.jmedchem.4c00630

[86] Jochmans D, van Nieuwkoop S, Smits S, Neyts J, Fouchier R, Van Den Hoogen B. Antiviral activity of favipiravir (T-705) against a broad range of paramyxoviruses in vitro and against human metapneumovirus in hamsters. Antimicrobial Agents and Chemotherapy. 2016;**60**(8):4620-4629. DOI: 10.1128/AAC.00709-16

[87] Smyk JM, Majewska A. Favipiravir in the battle with respiratory viruses. Mini Reviews in Medicinal Chemistry. 2022;**22**(17):2224-2236. DOI: 10.2174/1389557522666220218122744

[88] Cox R, Plemper RK. The paramyxovirus polymerase complex as a target for next-generation anti-paramyxovirus therapeutics. Frontiers in Microbiology. 2015;**6**:459. DOI: 10.3389/fmicb.2015.00459

[89] Piacentini S, La Frazia S, Riccio A, Pedersen JZ, Topai A, Nicolotti O, et al. Nitazoxanide inhibits paramyxovirus replication by targeting the fusion protein folding: Role of glycoprotein-specific thiol oxidoreductase ERp57. Scientific Reports. 2018;**8**(1):10425. DOI: 10.1038/s41598-018-28172-9

[90] Farrukee R, Ait-Goughoulte M, Saunders PM, Londrigan SL, Reading PC. Host cell restriction factors of paramyxoviruses and pneumoviruses. Viruses. 2020;**12**(12):1381. DOI: 10.3390/v12121381

[91] Freed EO, Gale M Jr. Antiviral innate immunity: Editorial overview. Journal of Molecular Biology. 2014;**426**(6):1129. DOI: 10.1016/j.jmb.2014.01.005

[92] Wang C, Wang T, Duan L, Chen H, Hu R, Wang X, et al. Evasion of host antiviral innate immunity by paramyxovirus accessory proteins. Frontiers in Microbiology. 2022;**12**:790191. DOI: 10.3389/fmicb.2021.790191

[93] Bhol NK, Bhanjadeo MM, Singh AK, Dash UC, Ojha RR, Majhi S, et al. The interplay between cytokines, inflammation, and antioxidants: Mechanistic insights and therapeutic potentials of various antioxidants and anti-cytokine compounds. Biomedicine and Pharmacotherapy. 2024;**178**:117177. DOI: 10.1016/j.biopha.2024.117177

Section 3

Viral Replication and Production and Regulation

Chapter 5

The Role of Fibroblast Growth Factors in Viral Replication: FGF-2 as a Key Player

Danial Zareh, Reyhaneh Nekounam Ghadirli, Zuo Hao, Giti Paimard and Tahereh Alinejad

Abstract

Fibroblast growth factors (FGFs) are crucial signaling proteins that govern numerous cellular activities, such as proliferation, differentiation, and tissue repair. Recent studies indicate that FGFs, particularly FGF-2, are pivotal in viral replication by altering the host cell environment to promote viral survival, replication, and immune evasion. Viruses rely on host cell components for their replication and often manipulate host signaling pathways, including FGF signaling, to optimize their environment for viral growth. Among the various FGFs, FGF-2 (basic FGF) stands out as particularly influential in viral replication due to its roles in angiogenesis, cell survival, and immune modulation. This chapter explores the molecular processes via which various FGFs affect viral life cycles, particularly highlighting FGF-2, which is notably important in promoting viral replication via its impact on cell survival, angiogenesis, and inflammation. Understanding FGF-mediated viral replication may offer new therapeutic targets for viral infections.

Keywords: fibroblast growth factors, viral replication, antiviral therapy, FGF-2, cell survival, angiogenesis, inflammation

1. Introduction

Broad-spectrum mitogens called fibroblast growth factors (FGFs) control cellular processes, such as migration, proliferation, differentiation, and survival. FGF signaling is crucial for tissue homeostasis, metabolism, and development. Numerous human disorders, including congenital craniosynostosis and dwarfism syndromes, chronic kidney disease (CKD), obesity, insulin resistance, and several types of malignancies, are linked to the FGF/FGF receptor (FGFR) signaling axis dysfunction [1].

One of the most varied families of growth factors in vertebrates is the FGF family. There are 22 known FGF ligands in both humans and mice. The 18 canonical mammalian FGFs are separated into six subfamilies, comprising one endocrine subfamily and five paracrine subfamilies, based on phylogeny and sequence homology. FGF1 subfamily (FGF1 and FGF2), FGF4 subfamily (FGF4, FGF5, and FGF6), FGF7 subfamily (FGF3, FGF7, FGF10, and FGF22), FGF8 subfamily (FGF8, FGF17, and FGF18), and FGF9 subfamily (FGF9, FGF16, and FGF20) are the five paracrine subfamilies. Endocrine signals are produced by the FGF19 subfamily, which includes FGF19, FGF21, and FGF23 [2].

By binding and activating high-affinity tyrosine kinase receptors encoded by four genes (FGFR1, FGFR2, FGFR3, and FGFR4) as well as FGFRL1, a shortened form of FGFR without an intracellular domain, in mammals, FGFs produce their pleiotropic effects. FGFRs are single-pass transmembrane proteins with an intracellular tyrosine kinase domain, an extracellular domain, and a transmembrane domain (TMD). Three immunoglobulin (Ig)-like domains (D1–D3), an acidic area, a heparin-binding motif for FGFs, heparan cofactors, and partner proteins make up the extracellular domain. The TMD helps the receptors dimerize and anchor them in the cell membrane. While the split kinase domains are necessary for the transmission of FGF-related signals, the juxtamembrane region of FGFRs plays a role in receptor dimerization in the cytosol [3, 4].

As previously stated, a class of proteins known as fibroblast growth factors (FGFs) is essential for the growth and upkeep of many bodily tissues. FGFs fall into three functional groups: intracellularly retained FGFs, metabolic (also known as endocrine) FGFs, and canonical FGFs (cFGFs). Secreted and acting in an autocrine/paracrine manner, cFGFs control tissue healing in adults and differentiation during fetal development. FGF-2 and other canonical FGFs may play a significant virus-specific role via regulating the immune response, according to recent research that has started to clarify the function of cFGFs during viral infections. Many anticancer medications target FGFs because instability in the FGF pathways plays a crucial role in the development of cancer. Since the pathophysiology of viral infections, including hepatitis C, has been linked to dysregulation of FGF signaling, these medications may be repurposed to treat viral infections. In general, there is currently a dearth of studies on the function of cFGFs during viral infection [5].

2. cFGFs or canonical FGFs

Heparan sulfates (HS) encapsulate cFGFs on the extracellular matrix (EM) and shield them from protease digestion. Despite binding their FGF receptors (FGFRs), they stay connected to HS because they are necessary for FGFR binding and activation [6, 7].

FGF binding proteins and HS can both tune expression, secretion, and retention to positively regulate FGF activity [8]. In fact, research is being done on these FGF-trapping compounds as potential new cancer treatments [9]. FGF availability can also be controlled by processing FGFR into soluble FGF traps that compete with membrane-bound FGFR or by dimerization, as explained for FGF9. Numerous mechanisms influencing FGFR internalization can further modulate FGF activity [8]. The FGF pathway is a difficult system to research and comprehend because of its complexity and the different regulatory mechanisms that influence its activity.

Every canonical FGF has a significant function in ontogenesis [8]. Nonetheless, the most often researched cFGFs during viral infection consist of:

1. Acid FGF, or FGF1. All FGFRs can be bound by FGF1 [2].

2. FGF2, commonly referred to as basic FGF, phosphorylates ERK1/2 and performs many of the same tasks as FGF1. Only the lightest of the four FGF2 isoforms is released; the heavier isoforms act in the cells where they are generated. Phosphatidylinositol 4,5-bisphosphate (PI(4,5)P2) on the inner leaflet of the plasma

membrane and heparan sulfates (HS) on the outer leaflet, where it binds to HS, are necessary for the special ER-independent mechanism that secretes FGF2. Compared to FGF1, FGF2 is more stable [10–12].

3. Two isoforms of FGF4 have conflicting functions: isoform 2 prevents isoform 1-induced Erk1/2 phosphorylation. Isoform 2 of FGF4 is still expressed after differentiation, whereas isoform 1 is no longer expressed in differentiated cells [8].

4. Because it solely stimulates FGFR2b, which is found in keratinocytes, FGF7 is often referred to as keratinocyte growth factor (KGF).

5. Members of the FGF9 subfamily are inactive dimers that are attached to HS. Since FGFRs can only be bound by monomers, dimerization is a crucial regulation mechanism for this family [8].

6. FGFR2b is also bound by FGF10, commonly referred to as keratinocyte growth factor 2 (KGF2). Given that lipopolysaccharides (LPS) have been demonstrated to downregulate FGF10 expression, it might be involved in lung inflammation. However, FGF10's role in inflammation is not unique; FGF7 and FGF2 have also been linked to this phenomenon [13].

3. FGFR localization and structure

Four genes, Fgfr1-4, encode the membrane tyrosine kinases (TKs) known as FGFRs. The three extracellular immunoglobulin-like domains (IGLD) that make up FGFRs—I, II, and III—bind HS and FGFs. Together with IGLD-I, the acidic box that connects the external IGLD-I and -II functions as an autoinhibitory regulator of FGFR [14]. Two successive intracellular TK domains, −1 and −2, which bind ATP and its phosphorylation substrates, are connected to the IGLD-III by a transmembrane domain [8].

While FGFR4 is a single receptor, the mRNAs for FGFR-1, −2, and − 3 can alternatively splice to produce mutually exclusive IGLD III variants, known as -b and -c. FGFR-1b, −1c, −2b, −2c, −3b, −3c, and −4 are seven possible FGFR variations that have varying tissue expression patterns, FGF-binding specificities, and affinities. Mesenchymal cells exhibit the -c variations, whereas epithelial cells express the -b versions [8].

It is believed that FGFR-like 1, the eighth member of the FGFR family, binds at least part of the FGFs that are secreted. FGFR-like 1 has a short intracellular tail with an odd histidine-rich pattern, but it does not have the TK domain. Some of the functions of FGFs are counteracted by it [15].

3.1 The process of signaling by FGFR

Numerous mechanisms, including sequestration of released FGF on the EM, regulation of FGFR synthesis, splice variants, and FGFs, govern FGF activity [8]. The recruitment of various cofactors by FGFRs, which modifies the impact of ligand-receptor interaction and diversifies the result of FGFR activation, is another method of controlling FGF activity. A number of regulators, including the intracellular negative regulator of receptor TKs Sprouty 1-2-4, are also involved in the negative control of FGFR signaling [16].

Trimeric HS-FGF-FGFR complexes are created when cFGF binds to FGFRs on the cell surface, and these complexes are then endocytosed. The FGFR is autophosphorylated by its TK domains in the cytoplasm, which attracts cellular cofactors. Following phosphorylation, four pathways may then be activated.

1. PLCγ, or phospholipase Cγ. The phosphorylated tyrosine residue (P-Tyr)-766 is the unique binding site for PLCγ. It produces two-second messengers, inositol 1,4,5-trisphosphate (IP3) and diacylglycerol (DAG), when it breaks down phosphatidylinositol 4,5-bisphosphate (PI(4,5)P2; PIP2) in lipid vesicles. While DAG attracts and activates protein kinase C on the membrane, IP3 binds to receptors on the ER, releasing calcium ions (Ca2+) into the cytoplasm [17].

2. Nuclear translocation of the transcription factors STAT-1, −3, and −5. The proteins STAT 3 and 5 are essential for inflammation and the body's reaction to cytokines, and they are frequently implicated in the development of cancer. In addition to its primary tumor-suppressive and perhaps antiviral properties, STAT1 is anti-apoptotic and participates in the IFN pathways [1].

3. The MPK/ERK circuit FRS2α plays a crucial part in the activation of the Ras/Mitogen-activated protein (MAP)-K (sometimes referred to as the Ras-Raf-MEK-ERK) pathway. The intracellular domain of FGFR is constitutively linked to this docking protein. A kinase cascade, comprising serine/threonine kinases such AR-AF/BRAF/CRAF, the dual specificity kinase MEK1/2, and the serine/threonine kinases ERK1/2, may be triggered by its association with other proteins [18].

4. When FRS2α binds to the GAB1 protein, the PI3K-Akt signaling pathway is activated [19].

3.2 FGFR activation effects

Cell death inhibition, dedifferentiation, and proliferation.

FGFs are still utilized in biological experiments for this purpose because they were found to have the capacity to promote DNA synthesis and fibroblast proliferation [20]. FGFs also prolong the longevity of endothelial cells and fibroblasts by preventing senescence and death. By preserving the expression of transcription factors that control stemness, they also inhibit the development of vascular smooth muscle cells and keratinocytes. In cell culture, FGFs (particularly FGF2) are added to the culture medium of keratinocytes and embryonic stem cells in order to take advantage of their capacity to preserve cell stemness [21]. Although it plays a role in the pathophysiology of atherosclerosis and is a major factor in the induction of cancer, FGFs can also encourage the dedifferentiation of various cell types, which is advantageous for tissue repair. Mutations in the genes encoding FGF and its receptors are frequently detected in some cancer types [17, 22]. Additionally, research conducted in vivo has demonstrated that FGFs aid in the healing of wounds in higher vertebrates [23, 24].

It is interesting to note that cells activated by FGF1, FGF2, or FGF9 will revert to quiescence if FGF is taken away. Different cell types experience a refractory phase, also known as FGF memory, during which they are unable to respond to FGF stimulation. This is an epigenetic process that is dependent on the production of IL1α and NFκB signaling [25].

Tissue repair and EM remodeling: damage to the tissue causes inflammation and HS cleavage in EM. In addition to the cFGF released by immune cells during the process, this makes cFGFs available for tissue repair. As demonstrated by transcriptome analysis for human fibroblasts, where expression of metalloproteinases, which are a component of the EM, was markedly elevated with FGF2 treatment, cFGFs in turn aid in the accumulation of EM [26].

Fibrosis and tissue regeneration: Fibrosis is a normal tissue-healing process in which scarring tissue, collagen, and fibroblasts repair injured tissue. Fibrosis is necessary for tissue repair, but too much or prolonged fibrosis can seriously impair organ function. Cirrhosis, liver failure, and an elevated risk of hepatocellular cancer are all consequences of increasing fibrosis in the liver [27].

Inflammation: FGF signaling's role in inflammation has been extensively researched, and data indicates that it can influence cytokine synthesis and function as well as encourage immune cell migration, including that of macrophages (MF), to inflammatory tissues [13, 28, 29].

By interacting with resident tissue cells, MFs play a critical role in inflammation and aid in tissue remodeling and pathogenesis. The differentiation of monocytes and resident MFs into different functional phenotypes can be influenced by soluble factors such as cytokines; M1 MFs mainly promote inflammation, while M2 MFs stimulate healing and reduce inflammation [30].

On the other hand, it has been demonstrated that FGFR1 phosphorylates NFκB, activating it and causing inflammation. Furthermore, it has been demonstrated that FGF7 and FGF10 promote the synthesis of proinflammatory cytokines in a number of organs [13, 22]. Rheumatoid arthritis and inflammatory bowel disease are two chronic inflammatory diseases that have been connected to the dysregulation of FGF signaling [13, 31].

3.3 FGFs and viral infection

3.3.1 Insect viruses

Enveloped viruses use virus-encoded glycoproteins that promote membrane fusion to attach to cell surface receptors and penetrate target cells in order to infect their host. Once the virus envelope has fused with the endosomal or plasma membrane of the cell, the viral DNA is transferred into the cytoplasm for transcription and replication. Certain viruses, including influenza and lentiviruses, need to move their genome to the nucleus to replicate.

Advanced programs are installed in cells to fight off viral infections. Antiviral signaling cascades downstream of ligand-activated receptors are part of these programs. Numerous ligands that are secreted either locally or systemically exhibit antiviral properties [32].

Certain viruses, including dsDNA viruses, such as Iridoviridae, herpesviruses, and poxviruses, include sequences that are similar to those in human cells [33]. These viruses can use their resemblance to mimic endogenous factors and produce growth factor homologs by taking advantage of host genes. These GF homologs then trigger pathways that support viral activities, such as cellular transformation, viral infection, and viral metabolic needs.

Numerous viruses include sequences that are very similar to human peptides, such as insulin, insulin-like growth factors (IGF)-1 and −2, fibroblast growth factor (FGF), and vascular endothelial growth factor (VEGF), according to a thorough bioinformatics-driven study. One of the most prevalent factors encoded by the virus family Iridoviridae is viral insulin/IGF-1-like peptides (VILPs) [33].

Since most viruses need an active environment to proliferate, they have developed ways to stimulate cell metabolism. This is especially true for viruses that cause cancer [34]. Since the FGF pathways give viruses a perfect means to increase cell metabolism, FGFs may be essential for viral replication but may also be the focus of other FGF effects. Interestingly, insect viruses that rely on FGF heavily—such as *Autographa californica* multiple nucleopolyhedrovirus—even have their own FGF (vFGF) gene, which is translated during viral replication. Since midgut epithelial cells are normally segregated by a basal lamina that hinders interaction with the underlying tissue, vFGF enables insect infections to reach other organs. According to the suggested process, metalloproteases in the EM are successively activated, triggering caspases that are transferred outside infected cells. By cleaving tracheal basal layer proteins, caspases allow infection to move throughout the body [35].

Although there is no evidence of vFGF for mammalian viruses, arboviruses that infect both mammals and insects have transmission difficulties comparable to those faced by insect viruses. To reach the salivary gland, they must also move systemically from the midgut, where the infected blood meal is administered. The main way that arthropods transmit and how humans contract arboviral infections is by saliva, a highly contagious bodily fluid. According to recent research, the Alphavirus Sindbis virus's capacity to reproduce in mosquitoes can be inhibited by lowering FGF signaling [36]. Perhaps because FGF secretion is already highly prevalent in infected mosquitoes, overexpression of FGF by a recombinant Sindbis virus had little effect. These results lend validity to the idea that FGF signaling is essential for arboviruses to spread through their arthropod vectors.

3.3.2 Human viruses and FGFs

As seen with HSV1-infected mouse brain neurons and ZIKA virus (ZIKV)-infected human primary astrocytes, which released FGF-4, −8, and −9, cells may release FGFs during infection to aid in recovery, similar to other types of tissue damage. Ironically, FGFs may also aid in the spread of viruses. Their ultimate influence is the "vectorial sum" of multiple potential processes, such as indirect effects on viral replication through the stimulation of cell proliferation or the IFN type I response. Furthermore, FGFs may have a variety of effects on viral pathogenicity in vivo, mostly through influencing immunological response and inflammation [37, 38].

Furthermore, viral replication is facilitated by interruption of IFN signaling caused by fibroblast growth factor (FGF). FGFs can stimulate the growth of several viruses, such as Zika, HSV-1, and lymphocytic choriomeningitis virus. FGF receptor kinase and proteasome activity are necessary for FGFs to have their transcriptional-level inhibitory effect on IFN-stimulated genes (ISGs) [39].

3.3.3 FGF2

Microcephaly and other neurological abnormalities in developing fetuses can be caused by the Zika virus (ZIKV), an emerging infection. Uncertainty surrounds the prenatal brain's biological reaction to ZIKV. The most prevalent cell type in the brain, human fetal astrocytes (HFAs) have been shown to produce and secrete more fibroblast growth factor 2 (FGF2) when infected with ZIKV. In human fetal brain explants and HFAs, this cytokine has been demonstrated to promote ZIKV replication and dissemination. Suppression of the interferon response is probably one of the ways that FGF2 has a proviral effect. This is a new way that viruses counteract host antiviral defenses [37].

It was recently discovered that Sertoli cells infected with ZIKV have significantly higher levels of FGF2 [40]. Furthermore, Limonta et al. showed that astrocytes released FGF2 in response to ZIKV infection, with this release peaking 48 hours after infection. Consequently, FGF2 suppressed the IFN type I response and enhanced ZIKV replication by activating MAP kinase [37]. Remarkably, the more pathogenic Asian strains of ZIKV, Brazil, and PRVABC-59, which caused the current microcephaly outbreaks in the Pacific Islands, were more successful in stimulating FGF2 release than the African strain [41]. In this context, it has been hypothesized that substantial alterations in ZIKV have caused the virus to evolve from a moderate illness to a serious cause of microcephaly; one such change may be an increased capacity to trigger FGF release. According to Kam et al., acute-phase ZIKV-infected individuals exhibited increased serum levels of FGF2 and other mediators that led to NFκB activation [42], which supports the idea that FGF plays a role in ZIKV pathogenicity. Nevertheless, during influenza, FGF2 was also found to be upregulated in mouse and patient sera, where it encouraged the recruitment of neutrophils [43]. It also indicates that ZIKV infections may not be the exclusive cause of FGF release.

In other studies, ZIKV-infected mouse keratinocytes, epithelial cells, or a human colon cancer line were treated with the keratinocyte growth factors FGF-7 or −10. IFN type I-stimulated genes were suppressed as a result of treatment [39]. The FGFR2b splice variation, the major keratinocyte growth factor receptor, was responsible for this result. It binds to FGF2 poorly by MEK1/2, PI3K, and/or the proteasome, but not by PLCγ. Keratinocytes treated with FGF exhibited increased HSV1, ZIKV, and LCMV multiplication. As a result, although through various FGFRs and signaling pathways, distinct FGFs enhance viral proliferation. Glial activation was discovered to be "switched on" by FGFs in the research where HSV1 infection of mouse neurons and astrocytes increased the synthesis of FGF-4, 8-, and -9. It is interesting to note that this effect was achieved in conjunction with the ubiquitin ligase HSV1 ICP0 protein, indicating that viruses may manipulate FGF's effects to their benefit [38]. In this regard, we have recently reported that ZIKV infection modifies nuclear localization and the transcription factor Forkhead box g1 (FOXG1) levels, leading to its down-regulation and export from the nucleus [44]. This effect may be a contributing factor to microcephaly, as FOXG1 is necessary for the development of the telencephalon in all animals [45]. When given to cells before infection, growth factors like EGF and FGF2 prevented ZIKV-mediated FOXG1 nuclear export and contributed to FOXG1 downregulation after ZIKV infection. The results reveal that FGF may contribute to pathogenesis in a very specific manner, namely by collaborating with viral proteins, given the effect on FOXG1 was unique to ZIKV. Given this, the PI3K-AKT pathway, one of the four pathways activated by FGFs, which is involved in the export mechanism of FOXG1 from the nucleus, may be crucial, as evidenced by several ZIKV impacts on cells [46, 47].

EGFR or PDGFR are said to be the most prevalent GFs used to control virus replication in SARS-CoV-2 infection. Patients with idiopathic pulmonary fibrosis can avoid fibrosis and viral replication by inhibiting GF downstream signaling [48]. Furthermore, dysregulated expression of various GFs, including VEGF, PDGF, IGF-1, and TGF-β, has been linked to several problems in SARS-CoV-2 infected patients, including coagulopathy; however, the precise mechanism by which the GFs exert these co-pathologies is yet unknown [49]. Additionally, there was a high correlation found between the severity of the disease and the expression of PDGF and FGF-2 [50].

3.4 Viral exploitation of FGFs and potential therapeutic targets

As previously noted, FGF signaling plays a crucial role in processes such as cellular proliferation, angiogenesis, differentiation, as well as tissue repair. These effects are beneficial but may provide a pro-survival and pro-growth microenvironment that can be virally exploited. Furthermore, FGFs are not directly involved in the immune response against infections but rather serve to repair damaged tissue [13, 28]. FGF has been studied as a potential therapeutic target in viral microenvironments as numerous viruses can utilize this pathway to replicate, propagate, and evade the host immune system [20].

Kaner et al. proposed that herpes simplex virus 1 (HSV-1) exploits FGF receptors (FGFR) to gain access to vertebrate cells and replicate. The results showed that Chinese hamster ovary cells that did not express the FGFR prevented viral entry and were resistant to HSV-1. Conversely, Chinese hamster ovary cells that were transfected with a complementary DNA that encoded a basic FGFR allowed viral entry and propagation to take place [51].

One of the neurological complications of HSV-1 infections is HSV-1 encephalitis (HSE). HSE can lead to severe damage and long-term neurological deficits [52, 53]. Glial cells that become activated during HSE secrete a variety of neurotrophic factors including FGF which promotes neuronal survival, axonal repair, and angiogenesis [54]. Hensel et al. showed that HSV-1 infected cortical cells of neonatal mice upregulated the expression of several FGFs and triggered paracrine FGF response. The results also showed the importance of ICP0, an *early viral protein* that is produced by HSV-1, in the transactivation of the host FGF system. This FGF response likely augments cell survival during infection and promotes tissue repair processes which would sustain host viability for HSV-1. These findings remain rather inconclusive and future studies need to be conducted to shed light on whether this is beneficial or if it facilitates viral spread in the context of HSV-1 [38].

Kaposi's sarcoma (KS) is an angiogenic tumor that is frequently found in human immunodeficiency virus-1 infected individuals and is caused by Kaposi's sarcoma-associated herpesvirus or human herpesvirus-8 (HHV-8). One study showed that the angiogenic FGF-2 and the Tat protein of HIV-1 were both expressed in KS lesions of HIV-infected patients and synergistically induced angiogenic KS-like lesions in mice [55].

Sgadari et al. showed that FGF-2 and HIV-1 Tat synergistically inhibit apoptosis via the upregulation of Bcl-2 expression in endothelial cells. Furthermore, FGF-2 and Tat activate pathways like the RAS/MAPK, thereby promoting proliferation and survival, as well as PI3K-AKT, thereby enhancing anti-apoptotic signals. FGF-2 further synergizes with TAT to upregulate integrin expression which promotes cell survival and adhesion [56]. FGF2 and TAT synergistically also increase telomerase activity in KS cells allowing them to proliferate indefinitely [57, 58]. This study provides insight into the therapeutic targets of this synergistic association and its link to Bcl-2 expression [58].

Epstein–Barr virus latent membrane protein 1 (LMP-1) has been shown to upregulate FGF-2 expression and lead to its extracellular release [59]. It has been proposed that this process is mediated by NF-κB signaling [60]. This released FGF-2 can lead to increased invasiveness of tumors, angiogenesis, and facilitate progression. Moreover, LMP-1 has been shown to promote FGF-2 release through exosomes [61]. This process involves the concentration of FGF-2 in vesicular bodies and its later release, which may play a role in enhancing the malignant microenvironment. It is important to note that studies have shown that NF-κB activation increases the expression of anti-apoptotic genes such as Bcl-2 and immunomodulatory molecules such as PD-L1 [62, 63]. These findings elucidate that LMP1-mediated modulation of FGF-2 and its link to Bcl-2 may be an important field for further exploration.

Preclinical studies have investigated the potential of Bcl-2 inhibitors in mitigating chronic viral infections characterized by apoptotic resistance, including HIV and EBV. These studies suggest that targeting Bcl-2 may enhance the elimination of infected cells. HIV-infected cells often exhibit increased expression of Bcl-2, contributing to the persistence of the virions. Inhibiting Bcl-2 can promote apoptosis and reduce the size of the viral reservoir [64, 65]. Venetoclax has also been shown to enhance immune effector functions and lead to decreased plasma viremia and reduced HIV reservoir size in humanized mouse models [65]. Combination therapy of bortezomib and venetoclax was shown to target the pro-survival protein Mcl-1 and Bcl-2 simultaneously in EBV-associated lymphoproliferative disorders, leading to the augmentation of apoptosis in these cells [66]. These findings are currently promising, but further in-depth research is necessary to fully understand the potential and safety of these Bcl-2 inhibitors in the context of chronic viral infections. FGFs are primarily involved in repair and regeneration and act like anti-apoptotic agents via their activation of survival pathways such as *PI3K/Akt* and *MAPK/ERK*, which have been shown to attenuate neuronal apoptosis [67]. The dual combinatorial use of FGFR inhibitors and Bcl-2 inhibitors has been explored in anti-cancer research. In one study, the FGFR-2 inhibitor (Dovitinib) and the BCL2 inhibitor (Venetoclax) were used in an FGFR-2 mutant endometrial cancer cell line, and this combination was shown to induce a synergistic effect on inducing mitochondrial-dependent apoptosis [68]. The use of Bcl-2 inhibitors as a form of adjunctive antiviral therapy in FGFR antiviral therapy is compelling and would be an interesting area to explore.

Virus-induced cancers such as Kaposi's sarcoma, Epstein–Barr virus-associated lymphomas, and human papillomavirus-associated cancers have been shown to frequently exhibit upregulated expression of Bcl-2 in EBV-associated lymphomas. Lu et al. showed that the viral latent membrane protein 1 (LMP-1) in human epithelial cells causes the expression of Bcl-2 *in vitro*, which leads to the inhibition of apoptosis and survival of infected B-cells. Furthermore, the co-expression of Bcl-2 and LMP-1 promotes the growth of epithelial cells *in vitro* [69]. In HPV-associated cancers, the viral oncoproteins E6 and E7 can lead to the upregulation of Bcl-2, thereby leading to the inhibition of apoptosis in infected cells [70, 71]. This overexpression or upregulation of Bcl-2 in these virus-induced malignant microenvironments highlights the potential of targeting Bcl-2 as a therapeutic strategy to promote apoptosis and augment the effectiveness of current treatments.

Blocking the interaction between FGF-2 and Tat or inhibiting downstream pathways involved in BCL-2 signaling could be a therapeutic strategy for mitigating the consequences of Kaposi's sarcoma. Furthermore, drugs that inhibit BCL2, such as venetoclax, may aid in the restoration of apoptosis. Combination therapy may be helpful by combining anti-FGF-2 agents with antiretroviral therapy or agents that target HHV-8. Venetoclax has been primarily used in hematologic cancers with BCL-2 overexpression. Research into its broader applications, encompassing viral infections, solid tumors, as well as virus-induced cancers like KS is still ongoing, limited, and inconclusive [66, 72, 73]. Virus-induced cancers often involve a multifactorial network of viral and host survival pathways, making BCL-2 or FGF-2 inhibition alone likely insufficient. There are also concerns regarding the quality of target specificity and the induction of apoptosis in normal cells leading to unintended and unwarranted immunological consequences.

3.5 Role of FGFR in augmentation of viral vector systems

Viral vectors have become indispensable in research, therapeutics, and vaccine development due to their efficiency in delivering genetic material into host cells. Their versatility encompasses numerous fields in medicine including potential antiviral therapy. Viral vectors still pose potential challenges in terms of their potential immunogenicity, imprecise targeting, off-target complications, and high cost in terms of widespread clinical use [74, 75]. The use of FGFR has been explored in the realm of adeno-associated viral vectors to enhance viral vector delivery and specificity.

Studies have proposed three cell receptors for AAV2 infection. The heparin sulfate proteoglycan (HSPG), the αVβ5 integrin, and FGFR-1 [76, 77]. The proteoglycan serves as a primary receptor while the other two serve as co-receptors. These studies underscore the role that FGFR1 plays in mediating the infection caused by AAV2 and offer therapeutic insights for pharmaceutical intervention and gene therapy interventions. Qing et al. proposed that non-permissive cells that lacked the FGFR1 could not be transduced by the virus unless the FGFR1 was expressed in these cells. They further showed that FGFR's role is unique since AAV infection did not take place in the presence of other receptors like EGFR. Furthermore, treatment with the basic fibroblast growth factor inhibited AAV2 infection and transduction in permissive cells, indicating that there may have been competitive binding between these two factors [78]. The understanding of FGFR as an essential receptor provides deeper insight into AAV2's tropism and entry. Gene therapy research in the future can utilize FGFR's and FGR1's role to design vectors with even higher specificity and enhanced efficacy.

High-affinity FGFRs are downregulated in normal tissues but upregulated in sites of tissue repair [20]. In a study conducted by Doukas et al., an FGF2-FAB chemical conjugate was created. The FAB antibody was bound to the adenoviral protein, and the FGF2 was chemically linked to the FAB fragment. This chemical conjugate allowed the adenovirus to bind to FGFR receptors and prevented its native tropism to the Coxsackie adenovirus receptor (CAR) and integrins, such as αVβ5. This retargeting enabled the adenovirus to bind to alternative and more specific receptors and prevent off-target effects such as non-target tissue toxicity. This strategy creates a bypass mechanism whereby the FGF2 retargeted vector bypasses the HSPG and instead interacts with the high-affinity FGFR. FGF2 retargeting is a significant research advancement and unlocks possibilities in viral vector engineering. This group of researchers also concluded that the internalization pathways such as receptor-mediated endocytosis, lysosomal processing, as well as ligand trafficking into the nucleus were more effective in FGF2-retargeted vectors than non-retargeted adenoviral vectors, and that this may be due to the extremely high affinity of FGFR which would facilitate robust ligand binding even at limited ligand concentrations. Moreover, it was shown that the number of FGFR receptors or the receptor density was not the sole governing reason for enhanced expression, further suggesting that there are intracellular mechanisms at play [79].

This study [79] addresses crucial limitations and could possibly pave the way to reducing the systemic side effects associated with vector systems and improving therapeutic results. It is important to note that further research is necessary to elucidate the mechanistic network involved in these processes. While initial *in vitro* and *in vivo* animal studies demonstrate promising results, it is important to have further extensive *in vivo* analysis in diverse animal models to further investigate these effects. Long-term safety studies are also imperative to objectively evaluate whether there is a long-term potential for adverse immune response to these chemically engineered conjugated ligands.

Murine leukemia virus vectors (MLV), the retroviral vector, have been extensively used in research and cancer gene therapy. MLV vectors are limited in their clinical use as they require actively dividing cells as a prerequisite for transduction [80]. They are potential promising candidates in clinical oncological therapy. MLV vectors have been replaced by lentiviral and adeno-associated viral systems due to this need for actively dividing cells but could be augmented and serve as a practical choice in specific areas due to its cost-effectiveness, stable integration capabilities, and genomic simplicity. MLV vectors also have comparatively lower immunogenicity, making them safe for repeated dosing [81].

Interestingly, one study aimed to overcome the limitation posed by MLV vectors *in vivo* by administering basic fibroblast growth factor (bFGF) or FGF2 exogenously to the adult rat brain to stimulate cell division in CNS cells, thus creating a fertile soil for MLV-mediated gene transfer. This exogenous administration of bFGF-induced cell division in the adult brain successfully, and the MLV-based gene transfer was significantly enhanced without requiring modifications to the MLV vector [82]. This study underscores the usefulness of growth factors in augmenting gene therapy strategies using MLV vectors particularly in tissues that have lower mitotic activities. These findings necessitate the need for future research in FGF co-treatment, engineering modifications, and evaluation of its safety in improving the MLV vector system and other vector systems. It is important to note that this supports the previous discussion regarding the role of FGF in enhancing host viability which can be exploited by viruses.

4. Interplay between SRC family kinases and FGFR inhibitors

SRC family kinases (SFKs), including Lyn kinase, play an essential role in cellular pathways involved in cell growth, migration, as well as differentiation. Lyn kinase, primarily recognized as a haemopoietic cell-specific kinase, has dual regulatory and modulatory mechanisms in B-cell receptor signaling. It can cause the induction of BCR signaling as well as also lead to the recruitment of inhibitory proteins to prevent over-exaggerated immune activation [83–85]. Notably, one study showed substantially diminished secretion of dengue and Zika virions, in non-hematopoietic cells upon inhibition of Lyn [86]. FGFR kinase inhibitors have been shown to have a promising broad-spectrum antiviral potential by specifically blocking the SFKs, particularly the Lyn kinase [87]. These kinases are critical mediators for numerous stages of the viral life cycle, including entry, propagation, and evasion [88].

The comprehensive study conducted by Stefanova et al., highlights the effectiveness against both RNA viruses, such as influenza and encephalomyocarditis virus (EMCV), as well as DNA viruses, such as HSV-1. FGFR inhibitors such as AZD4547 and BGJ398, used in oncology, have shown dose-dependent antiviral efficacy against HSV-1 in human primary keratinocytes *in vitro* and could be promising candidates to repurpose in antiviral therapy. Moreover, they observed the antiviral effects of AZD4547 and BGJ398 in HSV-1-infected intestinal epithelial cells. AZD4547 was also shown to possess suppressive effects in mouse embryonic fibroblasts infected with HSV-1 infection [87].

Mouse intestinal organoids infected with EMCV exhibited a notable reduction in viral RNA load in the presence of AZD4547. A significant reduction in infection was observed in both Huh7 and HeLa cell lines that were infected with the human coronavirus 229E (HCov229E). Furthermore, the Huh7 cell line infected with the influenza virus exhibited strong antiviral reduction by BGJ398, but slight reductions by AZD4547. This inference highlights the concept of tailored therapy and the necessity to select FGFR kinase inhibitors in accordance with the targeted cell type and viral agent. It was also concluded that AZD4547 and BGJ398 inhibit early stages of viral infection *in vitro* and that they exhibit effects that are less pronounced in post-viral exposure as opposed to prior exposure [87].

As previously noted, the antagonism of interferons by FGFs is yet another clinically notable issue to reiterate. FGFs antagonize interferon signaling through their transcriptional suppression of interferon-stimulated genes (ISGs), which are imperative in antiviral defense [39]. Stefanova et al. conducted RNA sequencing of the HaCaT keratinocyte cell line treated with AZD4547 and BGJ398 to evaluate the expression of genes that were affected by FGFR inhibitor treatment. The results showed an upregulation of ISGs such as RSAD2 and ISG15 in untreated cells, and a suppression of the same ISGs in *AZD4547* treated HSV-1 infected cells, despite a reduction in viral load. To further investigate these results, mimetics of RNA and DNA viruses were used, and the same effects were observed as in HSV-1 infected cells. These findings suggest that the antiviral effect of *AZD4547* is not due to upregulated ISG expression and that there may be other ISG-independent mechanisms involved. The ingenuity pathway analysis (IPA) showed a significant activation of pro-inflammatory and antiviral pathways. FGFR signaling was shown to reduce ERK1/2 and p38 phosphorylation which are important downstream signaling pathways in FGFR signaling, thereby confirming effective FGFR inhibition [87].

It was shown that FGFR inhibitors hindered viral replication and reduced the viral reservoir size in HaCat cells through the off-target inhibition of Lyn and other Src family kinases (SFKs). A correlation was observed between the antiviral activity of AZD4547 and the downregulation of Lyn phosphorylation at Tyr397, a crucial activation region. Decreased Lyn phosphorylation was also induced in primary human keratinocytes. A downstream target of Lyn kinase, annexin A2, also exhibited reduced phosphorylation with AZD4547 treatment [89]. Conversely, it was shown that other FGFR inhibitors such as BGJ398, Erdafitinib, and Debio-1347 did not significantly affect the activity of Lyn kinase. The results also showed that there was a synonymous antiviral effect upon reduction of Lyn activity in the presence of the pan-SFK inhibitor, AZD0530. This observation further consolidates the potential role of Lyn in antiviral reactions. Moreover, Roblitinib, an FGFR4 inhibitor did not possess any antiviral effects and did not alter Lyn activity [87].

Additionally, Lyn knockdown via siRNAs in HaCat cells was carried out to ascertain the role that Lyn plays. Results showed that there was a notably significant decrease in HSV-1 viral DNA in extracellular supernatants; however, results pertaining to intracellular viral load were more variable and less-pronounced. Furthermore, they suggested a key association between Lyn and AZD4547 as the activity of AZD4547 was markedly decreased in the Lyn knockdown cells [87]. FGFR inhibitors, particularly AZD4547, could be repurposed and used in combination therapy with preexisting antiviral and interferon therapies and aid in targeting pathways that are not currently addressed with preexistent antiviral therapies.

Further research is necessary to elucidate if similar mechanisms of Lyn inhibition are present in persistent chronic viral infections such as HIV or hepatitis which often involve persistent viral reservoirs. FGFR inhibitors provide a host-directed therapeutic approach that targets host proteins that are crucial for enabling viral replication. Host-directed therapy mitigates the risk of resistance, which is a common challenge in direct-acting antivirals [90, 91]. Lyn and other SFKs are imperative meditators for normal cellular processes, including immunological function. The selectivity of FGFR inhibitors must be further augmented for viral processes without impacting essential host cellular functions via off-target interactions.

5. Host-directed therapy and potential viral resistance

It is less plausible that viruses could gain resistance in host-directed therapy and adapt to these alterations in host signaling, but as described in the literature it could still be a possibility [92]. This highlights the need for the utility of combination therapies or other strategies to mitigate the risks of viral resistance. It is noteworthy to mention that SFKs such as Lyn have been shown to be overexpressed in Kaposi's sarcoma via interactions with the associated herpesvirus K1 protein [93]. These FGFR inhibitors could potentially play a dual role by being active against the virus as well as the associated viral oncogenic processes that upregulate these kinases. These preclinical findings need to be validated in further clinical trials to assess its safety, efficacy, and optimal dosage in the long run.

Numerous findings from several studies are probably medically significant because they recommend the use of FGFR inhibitors to treat viral infections in people. Most likely, such a method would not be limited to the skin. According to this theory, FGF2 stimulated the generation of hepatitis C virion in hepatoma cells [94] and human fetal astrocytes infected with the Zika virus [37]. Additionally, FGF7 or FGF2 inhibited the expression of some ISGs in human astrocytes [37], colon cancer cells [95], or lung epithelial cells [95]. However, because FGFR inhibitors may interfere with tissue recovery, their use as an antiviral method will necessitate careful treatment timing. The healing of mouse lungs following influenza virus infection was hindered by suppression of FGFR signaling [96]. In addition to timing, the type of cell that is impacted and the way that FGFR is expressed by it is probably important. Therefore, through an as-yet-undiscovered mechanism that is independent of ISG regulation, a subset of FGFs, which primarily activate FGFR3, prevented infection of various cancer cell types with vesicular stomatitis virus or Coxsackie virus [32]. Thus, it will be crucial to ascertain whether FGFR inhibitors make some cancer cells more vulnerable to viruses rather than protecting them, as many of these cells exhibit dysregulated FGFR signaling [97]. Additionally, as demonstrated recently for the dengue virus, where inhibition of FGFR4 reduced viral replication but increased the infectivity of the resultant virions, other effects of FGFs on the viral life cycle must be taken into account [98]. Because FGFR kinase inhibitors, FGFR neutralizing antibodies, or FGF ligand traps are in clinical trials for the treatment of various cancer types and are generally well tolerated, the possibility of employing FGFR inhibition as an antiviral strategy is encouraging despite these unanswered questions [97, 99].

6. Adverse effects of FGFR inhibitors

While FGFR inhibitors have shown favorable results, their use is not without risks and adverse effects. FGF-1 inhibition interferes with FGF23 signaling, a regulator involved in the metabolism of phosphate, which can consequently lead to hyperphosphatemia [100, 101]. Hyperphosphatemia can problematically cause vascular calcifications, nephrological damage, as well as cardiovascular complications. It is therefore important to regularly monitor serum phosphate levels in patients using FGFR inhibitors. FGFR signaling is involved in the physiological turnover of epithelial cells in the gastrointestinal tract. Inhibition can trigger the disruption of GI homeostasis and result in nausea, vomiting, and diarrhea [101]. Chronically, such GI complications may lead to malnutrition as well as imbalances in electrolytes. FGFR inhibition may lead to the manifestation of ocular toxicity causing complications such as retinal detachment, corneal deposits, and blurred vision [102, 103]. Therefore, antiviral therapies that target FGFR would necessitate ophthalmological consultations.

FGFR inhibition can deregulate keratinocyte proliferation and differentiation and lead to inflammation of the oral mucosa, dryness, and other dermatological issues such as hand-foot syndrome [100, 104]. Lastly, off-target effects are also important to consider. First generation FGFR inhibitors can target the ATP binding site of other tyrosine kinases such as VEGFR, PDGFR, and EGFR, thereby leading to abnormal signaling [105, 106] It is noteworthy to mention that there has been great improvement in the development of FGFR inhibitors. While the first generation was ATP competitive and not highly specific. The third and fourth generations have enhanced specificity [106].

While these inhibitors have known and documented adverse effects, it is important to consider that most of these studies were conducted in cancer clinical trials. Moreover, many associated adverse effects can be prophylactically managed [107]. The doses and duration of therapy that would be used in viral infections would be considerably reduced than those used in cancer therapy, likely reducing the occurrence of adverse effects. It is important to weigh the risks against the benefits and carry out a thorough risk–benefit ratio assessment in the future.

7. Future perspective and conclusion

This is a rapidly evolving area in need of more thorough research. *In silico* docking studies can be particularly instrumental and have been leveraged in computational anti-cancer screening of potential natural FGFR inhibitors to find natural phenolic compounds that have inhibitory effects against FGFR receptors [108]. To our knowledge, there are no well-documented molecular docking studies dedicated to the screening of potential natural FGFR inhibitors in antiviral therapy. It is, therefore, necessary to bridge the gap in this area. In-depth research on dosage, administration method, effectiveness against various viruses, and adverse effects in virus-infected individuals will be necessary for such a novel indication for FGFR inhibitors. However, considering the limited alternatives for treating viral illnesses, some of which have a high fatality rate or for which vaccines are not yet available the endeavor appears to be worthwhile. Virostatic drugs are commonly used because they disrupt the viral life cycle. Nevertheless, they frequently show significant toxicity and are virus-specific, making them vulnerable to viral mutation. Therefore, there is an urgent need for better techniques, and FGFR inhibition may potentially provide a fundamentally different and up-and-coming strategy.

The results underscore the significance of FGF-2 in peripheral cells during viral replication, thus facilitating viral replication and immune evasion. Comprehending this facilitates the advancement of antiviral medicines to target FGF signaling pathways, potentially mitigating virus severity and enhancing patient outcomes. Future studies will clarify the exact molecular connections of FGF receptors and their replication mechanisms, particularly in viruses. Investigating the distinct functions of several FGFs in diverse illnesses can yield valuable insights. Moreover, the therapeutic potential of FGF enhancers, alongside their adverse effects and long-term effectiveness, will be essential in formulating targeted antiviral therapies.

Future perspectives include: (1) The investigation of the synergistic potential of FGF inhibitors in conjunction with current antiviral medications to enhance effectiveness and mitigate resistance development, (2) exploration of advanced drug delivery methods to target infected cells specifically, reducing the off-target effects of FGF inhibitors, (3) identification of biomarkers to forecast and assess the effectiveness of FGF-targeted therapy in viral suppression, and (4) the employment of synthetic biology techniques to engineer FGFs with altered characteristics that can function as decoys and interfere with therapeutic delivery mechanisms.

Author details

Danial Zareh[1], Reyhaneh Nekounam Ghadirli[2], Zuo Hao[3], Giti Paimard[4*] and Tahereh Alinejad[5*]

1 Faculty of Science, Department of Biology, University of Sistan and Baluchestan, Zahedan, Iran

2 Faculty of Medicine, Department of Pathophysiology, Medical University of Gdansk, Gdansk, Poland

3 Department of Gynecological Oncology and National Clinical Research Center for Obstetrics and Gynecology, Cancer Biology Research Center (Key Laboratory of the Ministry of Education), Tongji Hospital, Tongji Medical College, Huazhong University of Science and Technology, Wuhan, China

4 Laboratory of Novel Optoelectronic Technology for Ophthalmic Diagnostics (NOTOD), School of Ophthalmology and Optometry, School of Biomedical Engineering, State Key Laboratory of Ophthalmology Optometry, and Vision Science, Wenzhou Medical University, Wenzhou, Zhejiang, China

5 Institute of Cell Growth Factor, Oujiang Laboratory (Zhejiang Lab for Regenerative Medicine, Vision, and Brain Health), Wenzhou Medical University, Wenzhou, China

*Address all correspondence to: giti.paimard@gmail.com and talinejad698@gmail.com

References

[1] Xie Y, Su N, Yang J, Tan Q, Huang S, Jin M, et al. FGF/FGFR signaling in health and disease. Signal Transduction and Targeted Therapy. 2020;**5**(1):181. DOI: 10.1038/s41392-020-00222-7

[2] Ornitz DM, Itoh N. The fibroblast growth factor signaling pathway. Wiley Interdisciplinary Reviews: Developmental Biology. 2015;**4**(3):215-266. DOI: 10.1002/wdev.176. Epub 2015 Mar 13

[3] Wiedemann M, Trueb B. Characterization of a novel protein (FGFRL1) from human cartilage related to FGF receptors. Genomics. 2000;**69**(2):275-279. DOI: 10.1006/geno.2000.6332

[4] Goetz R, Mohammadi M. Exploring mechanisms of FGF signalling through the lens of structural biology. Nature Reviews. Molecular Cell Biology. 2013;**14**(3):166-180. DOI: 10.1038/nrm3528. Epub 2013 Feb 13

[5] Lottini G, Plicanti E, Lai M, Quaranta P, Pistello M, Freer G. Canonical fibroblast growth factors in viral infection. Reviews in Medical Virology. 2023;**33**(4):e2452. DOI: 10.1002/rmv.2452. Epub 2023 Apr 29

[6] Kang D, Jung SH, Lee GH, Lee S, Park HJ, Ko YG, et al. Sulfated syndecan 1 is critical to preventing cellular senescence by modulating fibroblast growth factor receptor endocytosis. The FASEB Journal. 2020;**34**(8):10316-10328. DOI: 10.1096/fj.201902714R. Epub 2020 Jun 12

[7] Weaver A, Bossaer JB. Fibroblast growth factor receptor (FGFR) inhibitors: A review of a novel therapeutic class. Journal of Oncology Pharmacy Practice. 2021;**27**(3):702-710. DOI: 10.1177/1078155220983425. Epub 2020 Dec 29

[8] Ornitz DM, Itoh N. New developments in the biology of fibroblast growth factors. WIREs Mechanisms of Disease. 2022;**14**(4):e1549. DOI: 10.1002/wsbm.1549. Epub 2022 Feb 9

[9] Presta M, Foglio E, Churruca Schuind A, Ronca R. Long pentraxin-3 modulates the angiogenic activity of fibroblast growth factor-2. Frontiers in Immunology. 2018;**9**:2327. DOI: 10.3389/fimmu.2018.02327

[10] Steringer JP, Lange S, Čujová S, Šachl R, Poojari C, Lolicato F, et al. Key steps in unconventional secretion of fibroblast growth factor 2 reconstituted with purified components. eLife. 2017;**6**:e28985. DOI: 10.7554/eLife.28985

[11] Koochaki R, Amini E, Zarehossini S, Zareh D, Haftcheshmeh SM, Jha SK, et al. Alkaloids in cancer therapy: Targeting the tumor microenvironment and metastasis signaling pathways. Fitoterapia. 2024;**179**:106222

[12] Lolicato F, Nickel W. A role for liquid-ordered plasma membrane nanodomains coordinating the unconventional secretory pathway of fibroblast growth factor 2? Frontiers in Cell and Development Biology. 2022;**10**:864257. DOI: 10.3389/fcell.2022.864257

[13] Marega M, Chen C, Bellusci S. Cross-talk between inflammation and fibroblast growth factor 10 during organogenesis and pathogenesis: Lessons learnt from the lung and other organs. Frontiers in Cell and Development Biology. 2021;**9**:656883. DOI: 10.3389/fcell.2021.656883

[14] Dai S, Zhou Z, Chen Z, Xu G, Chen Y. Fibroblast growth factor receptors (FGFRs): Structures and small molecule inhibitors. Cells. 2019;**8**(6):614. DOI: 10.3390/cells8060614

[15] Trueb B. Biology of FGFRL1, the fifth fibroblast growth factor receptor. Cellular and Molecular Life Sciences. 2011;**68**(6):951-964. DOI: 10.1007/s00018-010-0576-3. Epub 2010 Nov 16

[16] Wakioka T, Sasaki A, Kato R, Shouda T, Matsumoto A, Miyoshi K, et al. Spred is a sprouty-related suppressor of Ras signalling. Nature. 2001;**412**(6847):647-651. DOI: 10.1038/35088082

[17] Ferguson HR, Smith MP, Francavilla C. Fibroblast growth factor receptors (FGFRs) and noncanonical partners in cancer signaling. Cells. 2021;**10**(5):1201. DOI: 10.3390/cells10051201

[18] Pudewell S, Wittich C, Kazemein Jasemi NS, Bazgir F, Ahmadian MR. Accessory proteins of the RAS-MAPK pathway: Moving from the side line to the front line. Communications Biology. 2021;**4**(1):696. DOI: 10.1038/s42003-021-02149-3

[19] Hadari YR, Gotoh N, Kouhara H, Lax I, Schlessinger J. Critical role for the docking-protein FRS2 alpha in FGF receptor-mediated signal transduction pathways. Proceedings of the National Academy of Sciences of the United States of America. 2001;**98**(15):8578-8583. DOI: 10.1073/pnas.161259898. Epub 2001 Jul 10

[20] Maddaluno L, Urwyler C, Werner S. Fibroblast growth factors: Key players in regeneration and tissue repair. Development. 2017;**144**(22):4047-4060. DOI: 10.1242/dev.152587

[21] Lian AA, Yamaji Y, Kajiwara K, Takaki K, Mori H, Liew MWO, et al. A bioengineering approach for the development of fibroblast growth factor-7-functionalized sericin biomaterial applicable for the cultivation of keratinocytes. International Journal of Molecular Sciences. 2022;**23**(17):9953. DOI: 10.3390/ijms23179953

[22] Qi M, Xin S. FGF signaling contributes to atherosclerosis by enhancing the inflammatory response in vascular smooth muscle cells. Molecular Medicine Reports. 2019;**20**:162-170. Published online May 16

[23] Prudovsky I. Cellular mechanisms of FGF-stimulated tissue repair. Cells. 2021;**10**(7):1830. DOI: 10.3390/cells10071830

[24] Freiin von Hövel F, Kefalakes E, Grothe C. What can we learn from FGF-2 isoform-specific mouse mutants? Differential insights into FGF-2 physiology *in vivo*. International Journal of Molecular Sciences. 2020;**22**(1):390. DOI: 10.3390/ijms22010390

[25] Poole A, Kacer D, Cooper E, Tarantini F, Prudovsky I. Sustained inhibition of proliferative response after transient FGF stimulation is mediated by interleukin 1 signaling. Journal of Cellular Physiology. 2016;**231**(3):650-658. DOI: 10.1002/jcp.25111

[26] Kashpur O, LaPointe D, Ambady S, Ryder EF, Dominko T. FGF2-induced effects on transcriptome associated with regeneration competence in adult human fibroblasts. BMC Genomics. 2013;**14**:656. DOI: 10.1186/1471-2164-14-656

[27] Seitz T, Hellerbrand C. Role of fibroblast growth factor signalling in hepatic fibrosis. Liver International. 2021;**41**(6):1201-1215. DOI: 10.1111/liv.14863. Epub 2021 Mar 23

[28] Im JH, Buzzelli JN, Jones K, Franchini F, Gordon-Weeks A, Markelc B,

et al. FGF2 alters macrophage polarization, tumour immunity and growth and can be targeted during radiotherapy. Nature Communications. 2020;**11**(1):4064. DOI: 10.1038/s41467-020-17914-x

[29] Liang W, Wang Q, Ma H, Yan W, Yang J. Knockout of low molecular weight FGF2 attenuates atherosclerosis by reducing macrophage infiltration and oxidative stress in mice. Cellular Physiology and Biochemistry. 2018;**45**(4):1434-1443. DOI: 10.1159/000487569. Epub 2018 Feb 16

[30] Singla DK, Singla RD, Abdelli LS, Glass C. Fibroblast growth factor-9 enhances M2 macrophage differentiation and attenuates adverse cardiac remodeling in the infarcted diabetic heart. PLoS One. 2015;**10**(3):e0120739. DOI: 10.1371/journal.pone.0120739

[31] Shao X, Chen S, Yang D, Cao M, Yao Y, Wu Z, et al. FGF2 cooperates with IL-17 to promote autoimmune inflammation. Scientific Reports. 2017;**7**(1):7024. DOI: 10.1038/s41598-017-07597-8

[32] van Asten SD, Raaben M, Nota B, Spaapen RM. Secretome screening reveals fibroblast growth factors as novel inhibitors of viral replication. Journal of Virology. 2018;**92**(16):10-128

[33] Altindis E, Cai W, Sakaguchi M, Zhang F, Guo Xiao W, Liu F, et al. Viral insulin-like peptides activate human insulin and IGF-1 receptor signaling: A paradigm shift for host-microbe interactions. Proceedings of the National Academy of Sciences of the United States of America. 2018;**115**(10):2461-2466. DOI: 10.1073/pnas.1721117115. Epub 2018 Feb 21

[34] Purdy JG, Luftig MA. Reprogramming of cellular metabolic pathways by human oncogenic viruses. Current Opinion in Virology. 2019;**39**:60-69. DOI: 10.1016/j.coviro.2019.11.002. Epub 2019 Nov 22

[35] Means JC, Passarelli AL. Viral fibroblast growth factor, matrix metalloproteases, and caspases are associated with enhancing systemic infection by baculoviruses. Proceedings of the National Academy of Sciences of the United States of America. 2010;**107**(21):9825-9830. DOI: 10.1073/pnas.0913582107. Epub 2010 May 10

[36] Wu W, Simmons CA, Moffitt J, Clem RJ, Passarelli AL. Effects of manipulating fibroblast growth factor expression on sindbis virus replication *in vitro* and in *Aedes aegypti* mosquitoes. Viruses. 2020;**12**(9):943. DOI: 10.3390/v12090943

[37] Limonta D, Jovel J, Kumar A, Lu J, Hou S, Airo AM, et al. Fibroblast growth factor 2 enhances Zika virus infection in human fetal brain. The Journal of Infectious Diseases. 2019;**220**(8):1377-1387. DOI: 10.1093/infdis/jiz073

[38] Hensel N, Raker V, Förthmann B, Detering NT, Kubinski S, Buch A, et al. HSV-1 triggers paracrine fibroblast growth factor response from cortical brain cells via immediate-early protein ICP0. Journal of Neuroinflammation. 2019;**16**(1):248. DOI: 10.1186/s12974-019-1647-5

[39] Maddaluno L, Urwyler C, Rauschendorfer T, Meyer M, Stefanova D, Spörri R, et al. Antagonism of interferon signaling by fibroblast growth factors promotes viral replication. EMBO Molecular Medicine. 2020;**12**(9):e11793. DOI: 10.15252/emmm.201911793. Epub 2020 Jul 27

[40] Kumar A, Jovel J, Lopez-Orozco J, Limonta D, Airo AM, Hou S, et al. Human Sertoli cells support high levels of Zika virus replication and persistence.

Scientific Reports. 2018;**8**(1):5477. DOI: 10.1038/s41598-018-23899-x

[41] Hung SJ, Huang SW. Contributions of genetic evolution to zika virus emergence. Frontiers in Microbiology. 2021;**12**:12. DOI: 10.3389/fmicb.2021.655065

[42] Kam YW, Leite JA, Lum FM, Tan JJL, Lee B, Judice CC, et al. Specific biomarkers associated with neurological complications and congenital central nervous system abnormalities from zika virus-infected patients in Brazil. The Journal of Infectious Diseases. 2017;**216**(2):172-181. DOI: 10.1093/infdis/jix261

[43] Wang K, Lai C, Li T, Wang C, Wang W, Ni B, et al. Basic fibroblast growth factor protects against influenza A virus-induced acute lung injury by recruiting neutrophils. Journal of Molecular Cell Biology. 2018;**10**(6):573-585. DOI: 10.1093/jmcb/mjx047

[44] Lottini G, Baggiani M, Chesi G, D'Orsi B, Quaranta P, Lai M, et al. Zika virus induces FOXG1 nuclear displacement and downregulation in human neural progenitors. Stem Cell Reports. 2022;**17**(7):1683-1698. DOI: 10.1016/j.stemcr.2022.05.008. Epub 2022 Jun 16

[45] Mitter D, Pringsheim M, Kaulisch M, Plümacher KS, Schröder S, Warthemann R, et al. FOXG1 syndrome: Genotype-phenotype association in 83 patients with FOXG1 variants. Genetics in Medicine. 2018;**20**(1):98-108. DOI: 10.1038/gim.2017.75. Epub 2017 Jun 29

[46] Monel B, Compton AA, Bruel T, Amraoui S, Burlaud-Gaillard J, Roy N, et al. Zika virus induces massive cytoplasmic vacuolization and paraptosis-like death in infected cells. The EMBO Journal. 2017;**36**(12):1653-1668. DOI: 10.15252/embj.201695597. Epub 2017 May 4

[47] Liang Q, Luo Z, Zeng J, Chen W, Foo SS, Lee SA, et al. Zika virus NS4A and NS4B proteins deregulate Akt-mTOR signaling in human fetal neural stem cells to inhibit neurogenesis and induce autophagy. Cell Stem Cell. 2016;**19**(5):663-671. DOI: 10.1016/j.stem.2016.07.019. Epub 2016 Aug 11

[48] Klann K, Bojkova D, Tascher G, Ciesek S, Münch C, Cinatl J. Growth factor receptor signaling inhibition prevents SARS-CoV-2 replication. Molecular Cell. 2020;**80**(1):164-174.e4. DOI: 10.1016/j.molcel.2020.08.006. Epub 2020 Aug 11

[49] Ahmad F, Kannan M, Ansari AW. Role of SARS-CoV-2-induced cytokines and growth factors in coagulopathy and thromboembolism. Cytokine & Growth Factor Reviews. 2022;**63**:58-68

[50] Petrey AC, Qeadan F, Middleton EA, Pinchuk IV, Campbell RA, Beswick EJ. Cytokine release syndrome in COVID-19: Innate immune, vascular, and platelet pathogenic factors differ in severity of disease and sex. Journal of Leucocyte Biology. 2021;**109**(1):55-66

[51] Kaner RJ, Baird A, Mansukhani A, et al. Fibroblast growth factor receptor is a portal of cellular entry for herpes simplex virus type 1. Science. 1990;**248**(4961):1410-1413. DOI: 10.1126/science.2162560

[52] McGrath N, Anderson NE, Croxson MC, Powell KF. Herpes simplex encephalitis treated with acyclovir: Diagnosis and long term outcome. Journal of Neurology, Neurosurgery, and Psychiatry. 1997;**63**(3):321-326. DOI: 10.1136/jnnp.63.3.321

[53] Whitley RJ. Herpes simplex encephalitis: Adolescents and adults.

Antiviral Research. 2006;**71**(2-3):141-148. DOI: 10.1016/j.antiviral.2006.04.002

[54] Cui Q. Actions of neurotrophic factors and their signaling pathways in neuronal survival and axonal regeneration. Molecular Neurobiology. 2006;**33**(2):155-179. DOI: 10.1385/MN:33:2:155

[55] Ensoli B, Gendelman R, Markham P, et al. Synergy between basic fibroblast growth factor and HIV-1 tat protein in induction of Kaposi's sarcoma. Nature. 1994;**371**(6499):674-680. DOI: 10.1038/371674a0

[56] Barillari G, Sgadari C, Fiorelli V, et al. The tat protein of human immunodeficiency virus type-1 promotes vascular cell growth and locomotion by engaging the alpha5beta1 and alphavbeta3 integrins and by mobilizing sequestered basic fibroblast growth factor. Blood. 1999;**94**(2):663-672

[57] Barillari G, Franzese O, Comandini A, Bonmassar E, Ensoli B. Spindle cells from AIDS-associated Kaposi's sarcoma lesions express telomerase activity that is enhanced by Kaposi's sarcoma progression factors. Oncology Reports. 2010;**24**(1):219-223. DOI: 10.3892/or_00000849

[58] Sgadari C, Barillari G, Palladino C, et al. Fibroblast growth Factor-2 and the HIV-1 tat protein synergize in promoting Bcl-2 expression and preventing endothelial cell apoptosis: Implications for the pathogenesis of AIDS-associated Kaposi's sarcoma. International Journal of Vascular Medicine. 2011;**2011**:452729. DOI: 10.1155/2011/452729

[59] Finke J, Fritzen R, Ternes P, et al. Expression of bcl-2 in Burkitt's lymphoma cell lines: Induction by latent Epstein-Barr virus genes. Blood. 1992;**80**(2):459-469

[60] Wakisaka N, Murono S, Yoshizaki T, Furukawa M, Pagano JS. Epstein-Barr virus latent membrane protein 1 induces and causes release of fibroblast growth factor-2. Cancer Research. 2002;**62**(21):6337-6344

[61] Ceccarelli S, Visco V, Raffa S, Wakisaka N, Pagano JS, Torrisi MR. Epstein-Barr virus latent membrane protein 1 promotes concentration in multivesicular bodies of fibroblast growth factor 2 and its release through exosomes. International Journal of Cancer. 2007;**121**(7):1494-1506. DOI: 10.1002/ijc.22844

[62] Antonangeli F, Natalini A, Garassino MC, Sica A, Santoni A, Di Rosa F. Regulation of PD-L1 expression by NF-κB in cancer. Frontiers in Immunology. 2020;**11**:584626. Published 2020 Nov 25. DOI: 10.3389/fimmu.2020.584626

[63] Gerondakis S, Siebenlist U. Roles of the NF-kappaB pathway in lymphocyte development and function. Cold Spring Harbor Perspectives in Biology. 2010;**2**(5):a000182. DOI: 10.1101/cshperspect.a000182

[64] Chandrasekar AP, Cummins NW, Badley AD. The role of the BCL-2 family of proteins in HIV-1 pathogenesis and persistence. Clinical Microbiology Reviews. 2019;**33**(1):e00107-e00119. DOI: 10.1128/cmr.00107-19

[65] Chandrasekar AP, Cummins NW, Natesampillai S, et al. The BCL-2 inhibitor venetoclax augments immune effector function mediated by Fas ligand, TRAIL, and perforin/granzyme B, resulting in reduced plasma viremia and decreased HIV reservoir size during acute HIV infection in a humanized mouse model. Journal of Virology. 2022;**96**(23):e01730-e01722. DOI: 10.1128/jvi.01730-22

[66] Tam KP, Xie J, Au-Yeung RKH, Chiang AKS. Combination of bortezomib and venetoclax targets the pro-survival function of LMP-1 and EBNA-3C of Epstein-Barr virus in spontaneous lymphoblastoid cell lines. PLoS Pathogens. 2024;**20**(9):e1012250. DOI: 10.1371/journal.ppat.1012250. Published 2024 Sep 26

[67] Okada T, Enkhjargal B, Travis ZD, et al. FGF-2 attenuates neuronal apoptosis via FGFR3/PI3k/Akt signaling pathway after subarachnoid hemorrhage. Molecular Neurobiology. 2019;**56**(12):8203-8219. DOI: 10.1007/s12035-019-01668-9

[68] Packer LM, Stehbens SJ, Bonazzi VF, et al. Bcl-2 inhibitors enhance FGFR inhibitor-induced mitochondrial-dependent cell death in FGFR2-mutant endometrial cancer. Molecular Oncology. 2019;**13**(4):738-756. DOI: 10.1002/1878-0261.12422

[69] Lu JJ, Chen JY, Hsu TY, Yu WC, Su IJ, Yang CS. Cooperative interaction between Bcl-2 and Epstein-Barr virus latent membrane protein 1 in the growth transformation of human epithelial cells. The Journal of General Virology. 1997;**78**(Pt 11):2975-2985. DOI: 10.1099/0022-1317-78-11-2975

[70] Liang XH, Mungal S, Ayscue A, et al. Bcl-2 protooncogene expression in cervical carcinoma cell lines containing inactive p53. Journal of Cellular Biochemistry. 1995;**57**(3):509-521. DOI: 10.1002/jcb.240570316

[71] Alibek K, Irving S, Sautbayeva Z, et al. Disruption of Bcl-2 and Bcl-xL by viral proteins as a possible cause of cancer. Infect Agents Cancer. 2014;**9**:44. DOI: 10.1186/1750-9378-9-44

[72] Lindeman GJ, Fernando TM, Bowen R, et al. VERONICA: Randomized phase II study of fulvestrant and venetoclax in ER-positive metastatic breast cancer post-CDK4/6 inhibitors—Efficacy, safety, and biomarker results. Clinical Cancer Research. 2022;**28**(15):3256-3267. DOI: 10.1158/1078-0432.CCR-22-0260

[73] Ploumaki I, Triantafyllou E, Koumprentziotis IA, et al. Bcl-2 pathway inhibition in solid tumors: A review of clinical trials. Clinical & Translational Oncology. 2023;**25**:1554-1578. DOI: 10.1007/s12094-022-03070-9

[74] Waehler R, Russell SJ, Curiel DT. Engineering targeted viral vectors for gene therapy. Nature Reviews. Genetics. 2007;**8**(8):573-587. DOI: 10.1038/nrg2141

[75] Lundstrom K. Viral vectors in gene therapy: Where do we stand in 2023? Viruses. 2023;**15**(3):698. DOI: 10.3390/v15030698. Published 2023 Mar 7

[76] Summerford C, Samulski RJ. Membrane-associated heparan sulfate proteoglycan is a receptor for adeno-associated virus type 2 virions. Journal of Virology. 1998;**72**(2):1438-1445. DOI: 10.1128/JVI.72.2.1438-1445.1998

[77] Summerford C, Bartlett JS, Samulski RJ. Alpha Vbeta5 integrin: A co-receptor for adeno-associated virus type 2 infection. Nature Medicine. 1999;**5**(1):78-82. DOI: 10.1038/4768

[78] Qing K, Mah C, Hansen J, Zhou S, Dwarki V, Srivastava A. Human fibroblast growth factor receptor 1 is a co-receptor for infection by adeno-associated virus 2. Nature Medicine. 1999;**5**(1):71-77. DOI: 10.1038/4758

[79] Doukas J, Hoganson DK, Ong M, Ying W, Lacey DL, Baird A, et al. Retargeted delivery of adenoviral vectors through fibroblast growth factor receptors involves unique cellular pathways. The FASEB Journal.

1999;**13**(11):1459-1466. DOI: 10.1096/fasebj.13.11.1459

[80] Blesch A. Lentiviral and MLV based retroviral vectors for *ex vivo* and *in vivo* gene transfer. Methods. 2004;**33**(2):164-172. DOI: 10.1016/j.ymeth.2003.11.005

[81] Vargas JE, Chicaybam L, Stein RT, et al. Retroviral vectors and transposons for stable gene therapy: Advances, current challenges and perspectives. Journal of Translational Medicine. 2016;**14**:288. DOI: 10.1186/s12967-016-1047-x

[82] King LA, Mitrophanous KA, Clark LA, et al. Growth factor enhanced retroviral gene transfer to the adult central nervous system. Gene Therapy. 2000;7(13):1103-1111. DOI: 10.1038/sj.gt.3301198

[83] Yamanashi Y, Fukushige S, Semba K, et al. The yes-related cellular gene lyn encodes a possible tyrosine kinase similar to p56lck. Molecular and Cellular Biology. 1987;**7**(1):237-243. DOI: 10.1128/mcb.7.1.237-243.1987

[84] Ingley E. Functions of the Lyn tyrosine kinase in health and disease. Cell Communication and Signaling: CCS. 2012;**10**(1):21. DOI: 10.1186/1478-811X-10. Published 2012 Jul 17

[85] Xu Y, Harder KW, Huntington ND, Hibbs ML, Tarlinton DM. Lyn tyrosine kinase: Accentuating the positive and the negative. Immunity. 2005;**22**(1):9-18. DOI: 10.1016/j.immuni.2004.12.004

[86] Li MY, Naik TS, Siu LYL, et al. Lyn kinase regulates egress of flaviviruses in autophagosome-derived organelles. Nature Communications. 2020;**11**(1):5189. DOI: 10.1038/s41467-020-19028-w. Published 2020 Oct 15

[87] Stefanova D, Olszewski D, Glitscher M, et al. FGF receptor kinase inhibitors exhibit broad antiviral activity by targeting Src family kinases. Cellular and Molecular Life Sciences. 2024;**81**(1):471. DOI: 10.1007/s00018-024-05502-x. Published 2024 Dec 2

[88] Pagano MA, Tibaldi E, Palù G, Brunati AM. Viral proteins and Src family kinases: Mechanisms of pathogenicity from a "liaison dangereuse". World Journal of Virology. 2013;**2**(2):71-78. DOI: 10.5501/wjv.v2.i2.71

[89] Matsuda D, Nakayama Y, Horimoto S, et al. Involvement of Golgi-associated Lyn tyrosine kinase in the translocation of annexin II to the endoplasmic reticulum under oxidative stress. Experimental Cell Research. 2006;**312**(7):1205-1217. DOI: 10.1016/j.yexcr.2006.02.003

[90] Thom RE, D'Elia RV. Future applications of host direct therapies for infectious disease treatment. Frontiers in Immunology. 2024;**15**:1436557. DOI: 10.3389/fimmu.2024.1436557. Published 2024 Oct 1

[91] Bergman P, Raqib R, Rekha RS, Agerberth B, Gudmundsson GH. Host directed therapy against infection by boosting innate immunity. Frontiers in Immunology. 2020;**11**:1209. DOI: 10.3389/fimmu.2020.01209. Published 2020 Jun 12

[92] Kumar N, Sharma S, Kumar R, Tripathi BN, Barua S, Ly H, et al. Host-directed antiviral therapy. Clinical Microbiology Reviews. 2020;**33**(3):e00168-e00119. DOI: 10.1128/CMR.00168-19

[93] Prakash O, Swamy OR, Peng X, et al. Activation of Src kinase Lyn by the Kaposi sarcoma-associated herpesvirus K1 protein: Implications for lymphomagenesis. Blood. 2005;**105**(10):3987-3994. DOI: 10.1182/blood-2004-07-2781

[94] Van ND, Falk CS, Sandmann L, Vondran FW, Helfritz F, Wedemeyer H, et al. Modulation of HCV reinfection after orthotopic liver transplantation by fibroblast growth factor-2 and other non-interferon mediators. Gut. 2016;**65**:1015-1023

[95] Prince LS, Karp PH, Moninger TO, Welsh MJ. KGF alters gene expression in human airway epithelia: Potential regulation of the inflammatory response. Physiological Genomics. 2001;**6**:81-89

[96] Quantius J, Schmoldt C, Vazquez-Armendariz AI, Becker C, El Agha E, Wilhelm J, et al. Influenza virus infects epithelial stem/progenitor cells of the distal lung: Impact on Fgfr2b-driven epithelial repair. PLoS Pathogens. 2016;**12**:e1005544

[97] Tanner Y, Grose RP. Dysregulated FGF signalling in neoplastic disorders. Seminars in Cell and Developmental Biology. 2016;**53**:126-135

[98] Cortese M, Kumar A, Matula P, Kaderali L, Scaturro P, Erfle H, et al. Reciprocal effects of fibroblast growth factor receptor signaling on dengue virus replication and virion production. Cell Reports. 2019;**27**(2579-2592):e2576

[99] Touat M, Ileana E, Postel-Vinay S, Andre F, Soria JC. Targeting FGFR signaling in cancer. Clinical Cancer Research. 2015;**21**:2684-2694

[100] Loriot Y, Necchi A, Park SH, et al. Erdafitinib in locally advanced or metastatic urothelial carcinoma. The New England Journal of Medicine. 2019;**381**(4):338-348. DOI: 10.1056/NEJMoa1817323

[101] Javle M, Lowery M, Shroff RT, et al. Phase II study of BGJ398 in patients with FGFR-altered advanced cholangiocarcinoma. Journal of Clinical Oncology. 2018;**36**(3):276-282. DOI: 10.1200/JCO.2017.75.5009

[102] Furuse J, Goyal L, Meric-Bernstam F, et al. 116MO efficacy, safety, and quality of life (QoL) with futibatinib in patients (pts) with intrahepatic cholangiocarcinoma (iCCA) harboring FGFR2 fusions/rearrangements: FOENIX-CCA2. Annals of Oncology. 2020;**31**(Suppl. 4):S1288-S1289

[103] Hsu J, Francis JH, Ahmad S. Ocular toxicities of fibroblast growth factor receptor inhibitors: A review. Survey of Ophthalmology. 2024;**69**(1):34-41. DOI: 10.1016/j.survophthal.2023.09.007

[104] Kommalapati A, Tella SH, Borad M, Javle M, Mahipal A. FGFR inhibitors in oncology: Insight on the management of toxicities in clinical practice. Cancers. 2021;**13**(12):2968. DOI: 10.3390/cancers13122968

[105] Huang L, Jiang S, Shi Y. Tyrosine kinase inhibitors for solid tumors in the past 20 years (2001-2020). Journal of Hematology & Oncology. 2020;**13**(1):143. DOI: 10.1186/s13045-020-00977-0. Published 2020 Oct 27

[106] Zheng J, Zhang W, Li L, et al. Signaling pathway and small-molecule drug discovery of FGFR: A comprehensive review. Frontiers in Chemistry. 2022;**10**:860985. DOI: 10.3389/fchem.2022.860985

[107] Subbiah V, Verstovsek S. Clinical development and management of adverse events associated with FGFR inhibitors. Cell Reports Medicine. 2023;**4**(10):101204. DOI: 10.1016/j.xcrm.2023.101204

[108] Ekins S, Mestres J, Testa B. In silico pharmacology for drug discovery: Methods for virtual ligand screening and profiling. British Journal of Pharmacology. 2007;**152**(1):9-20. DOI: 10.1038/sj.bjp.0707305

Chapter 6

Viral Replication Regulated by Radiation

Yu Zhao, Yingyi Zhang, Yang Liu, Junling Zhang, Sen Wang, Danyue Qu, Xinyuan Ji and Saijun Fan

Abstract

Viruses are widely present in nature and can infect eukaryotic cells, producing a variety of biological effects. Several viruses are capable of coexisting with human cells over the long term, and it has been proven that these viruses possess carcinogenic properties. Radiation therapy is a common method used for treating tumors. Under the influence of radiation, infected tumor cells and uninfected tumor cells exhibit different pathological characteristics and treatment outcomes. Herein, in this chapter, we discuss the impact of five viruses on tumor radiation therapy, including coronavirus disease-2019 (COVID-19), hepatitis B virus (HBV), human papillomavirus (HPV), monkeypox virus, and avian influenza virus. We hope that by summarizing the relationship between viral replication and tumor radiation therapy, we can provide novel insight for future treatments.

Keywords: radiation therapy, COVID-19, HBV, HPV, monkeypox virus

1. Introduction

Viruses have a natural propensity to infect and replicate within cells, and certain viruses have shown a preference for tumor cells due to the altered metabolic and signaling pathways in these cells [1]. Oncolytic viruses, in particular, are engineered or naturally occurring viruses that selectively target and destroy cancer cells. They can directly lyse tumor cells, releasing viral particles and tumor antigens, which can further stimulate the host's immune system to mount an antitumor response [2]. The use of oncolytic viruses in cancer therapy is based on their ability to selectively infect and replicate within tumor cells, sparing normal cells. This selectivity is achieved through various mechanisms, including the exploitation of specific receptors on cancer cells, the activation of viral replication by tumor-specific promoters, and the enhancement of viral tropism for cancer cells [3]. Additionally, oncolytic viruses can be genetically modified to express therapeutic transgenes, further enhancing their antitumor effects [3].

The combination of viral infections and radiation therapy offers a synergistic approach to cancer treatment. Oncolytic viruses can enhance the effects of radiation in several ways: (1) Enhanced DNA damage: Oncolytic viruses can increase the sensitivity of cancer cells to radiation by disrupting the cell's DNA repair mechanisms [4]. This

IntechOpen

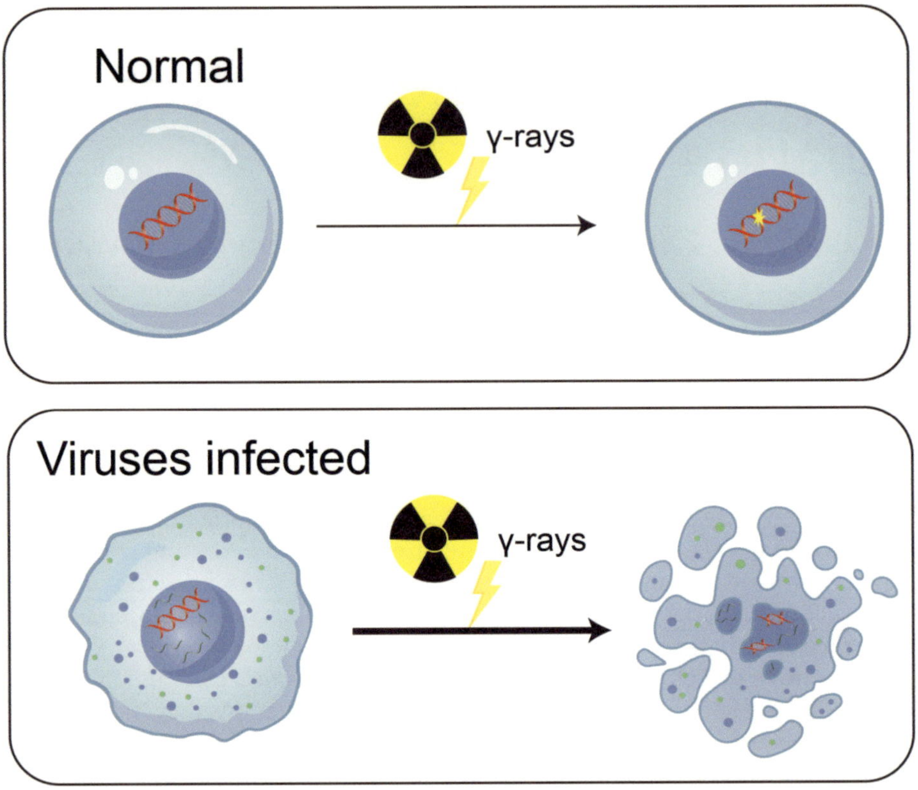

Figure 1.
Cancer cells infected with virus were sensitive to γ-radiation. Upper panel, the cell (blue) was treated with γ-radiation (yellow flash), the DNA (red) was damaged. Lower panel, the cell infected with virus (green), the DNA was damaged and cell was dead.

can lead to a more effective accumulation of DNA damage and an increased likelihood of cell death (**Figure 1**). (2) Immune activation: The lysis of cancer cells by oncolytic viruses releases tumor antigens, which can stimulate the host's immune system [5]. Radiation can also modulate the tumor microenvironment, making it more immunogenic. The combination of these two therapies can lead to a more robust antitumor-immune response. (3) Viral replication and spread: Radiation can create a more permissive environment for viral replication by inducing stress responses in cancer cells [3]. This can enhance the spread of oncolytic viruses within the tumor and increase the number of infected cells. (4) Overcoming resistance: Some cancer cells may develop resistance to either viral therapies or radiation. The combination of these two modalities can overcome such resistance by attacking the cancer cells through multiple pathways [6]. Thus, we summarize the combination effects of virus replications in cancer radiation therapies in the following sections.

2. COVID-19 virus

COVID-19, which is triggered by the novel coronavirus SARS-CoV-2, represents a respiratory infectious disease that first surfaced in Wuhan, China, toward the end of 2019. Ever since its initial eruption, this disease has been spreading at an alarming pace across the world, metamorphosing into one of the gravest public health emergencies in the twenty-first century. With its prominent features of a high transmission speed and potent infectivity, COVID-19 has cast a menacing shadow over global public health. In the arduous battle to forestall and govern the epidemic and, concurrently, to offer efficacious medical care to patients, radiological diagnostic and radiotherapeutic modalities have assumed a central position. These methodologies have, furthermore, emerged as the cynosure of copious research endeavors and clinical implementations. This part of chapter surveys the part that radiation plays in the diagnosis, administration, and treatment of COVID-19. It meticulously scrutinizes their clinical utilities, tackles the extant hurdles, and spotlights the prospective avenues for forthcoming research (**Figure 2**).

2.1 Radiological diagnostic for COVID-19 patients

2.1.1 Chest X-ray

Chest X-ray, as a traditional imaging method, remains an essential means for the initial screening of chest ailments. It can detect lung irregularities such as ground-glass opacities (GGOs) and consolidations, offering a rapid overview of the lungs. These abnormal features become observable because of the varying degrees of X-ray attenuation as they pass through human tissues, which then form images on film or digital detectors. Studies have indicated that chest X-ray can efficiently identify lung

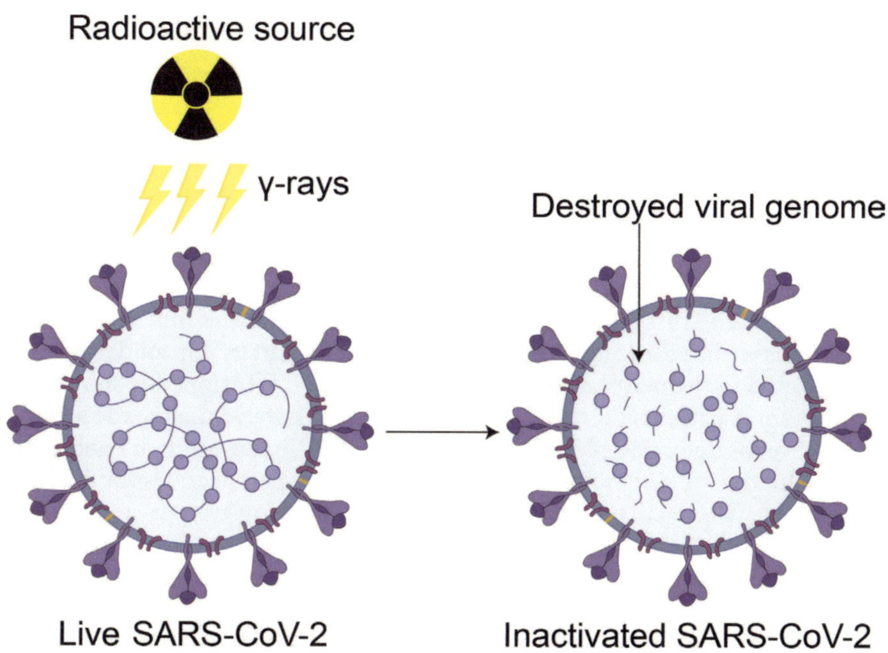

Figure 2.
Radio-ray destroyed the viral genomes. The SARS-CoV-2 genome is approximately 29.9 kb in length and contains a 5′ cap and a 3′ poly(A) tail, which are characteristic features of positive-sense RNA viruses (light purple line). The genome encodes a variety of structural and non-structural proteins (light purple cycles). The spike protein (dark purple) is a key target for vaccine development and therapeutic interventions. It undergoes conformational changes during viral entry, transitioning from a prefusion to a postfusion state. Post the radiation, the single-strand RNA was damaged.

involvement in patients at large-scale fever clinics, supplying valuable guidance for subsequent diagnostic steps [7, 8].

In patients with COVID-19, typical chest X-ray manifestations include bilateral, multifocal, and peripheral GGOs and consolidations, with the lesions predominantly concentrated in the lower lung regions [9, 10]. In severe cases, widespread bilateral lung consolidations might take place, resulting in the so-called "white lung" appearance. Given its speed, convenience, and ease of use, chest X-ray is particularly suitable for emergency and primary healthcare settings, allowing for its prompt application even in facilities with limited medical resources.

2.1.2 Computed tomography (CT)

CT, especially high-resolution computed tomography (HRCT), has been broadly recognized as the gold standard for diagnosing COVID-19 patients. It demonstrates high sensitivity and specificity, providing vital information that supports clinical decision-making and treatment planning [11–14]. In the initial phase of COVID-19, CT manifestations commonly present as bilateral, multifocal, and peripheral GGOs. As the illness progresses, more complex patterns, like consolidations, interstitial changes, and the so-called "crazy paving" pattern, may emerge. These lesions are often subpleural and mainly located in the basal lung regions [15]. However, the extremely high cost of CT equipment and the associated risks of radiation exposure limit its extensive use. When considering the application of CT, clinicians must carefully weigh multiple factors, such as the severity of the disease, the need for examination, and potential risks [16].

2.1.3 Ultrasound

Ultrasound imaging presents distinctive benefits when it comes to assessing pleural effusion, pulmonary consolidation, and cardiac function. It thereby serves as a significant adjunct to other imaging techniques. Typical pulmonary ultrasound manifestations in COVID-19 patients are as follows: (1) Augmented B-lines: These are comet-tail artifacts that stand perpendicular to the pleura and signify interstitial pulmonary edema. (2) Irregular pleural lines: Such irregularities hint at inflammatory alterations within the lung parenchyma. (3) Small, patchy consolidations: These are mostly found in the peripheral lung areas. (4) Pleural effusion: It is sporadically witnessed in some patients [17, 18]. Ultrasound has exhibited a diagnostic accuracy exceeding 95% for detecting pleural effusion [19, 20]. What is more, it enables the dynamic evaluation of cardiac function, offering crucial perspectives for the holistic management of COVID-19 patients.

2.1.4 Magnetic resonance imaging (MRI)

Although MRI is not frequently utilized in the routine diagnosis of COVID-19, it presents particular merits in specific circumstances: (1) Radiation-free: MRI eliminates ionizing radiation, which makes it highly preferable for patients who need repeated imaging scans, especially children and pregnant women. (2) Outstanding soft tissue contrast: MRI proves to be more efficacious than CT when it comes to evaluating soft tissue lesions and potential complications. (3) Multi-parametric imaging capabilities: MRI furnishes both functional and anatomical information, facilitating the evaluation of disease severity and predicting prognosis. Typical MRI manifestations in COVID-19 patients comprise high signal regions on T2-weighted images, corresponding to the GGOs and consolidations observable on CT. Abnormal signals detected on diffusion-weighted imaging (DWI) mirror the presence of inflammation and edema [21–24].

2.2 Radiotherapy for COVID-19 patients

At the commencement of the COVID-19 pandemic, the dearth of efficacious antiviral treatments impelled the medical fraternity to seek alternative therapeutic approaches. Among them, low-dose radiotherapy (LDRT) has garnered attention due to its prospective use in managing COVID-19-associated pneumonia [25, 26]. LDRT generally entails radiotherapy with doses lower than 1 Gray (Gy), and in the setting of COVID-19, it mainly focuses on the lungs, with dose magnitudes spanning from 0.5 to 1.5 Gy [27]. Several prospective studies have illustrated that LDRT is capable of substantially enhancing oxygenation indices in COVID-19 patients [28, 29]. Such enhancements are correlated with improved respiratory function, more favorable radiological imaging results, as well as decreases in inflammation-related biomarkers like C-reactive protein (CRP), interleukin-6 (IL-6), and lactate dehydrogenase (LDH) [28, 30, 31]. Moreover, it has been evidenced that LDRT can curtail hospitalization lengths, mitigate the 1-month mortality hazards, and prolong the survival spans for certain COVID-19 patients [29, 32]. The therapeutic effectiveness of LDRT is presumed to originate from its immunomodulatory features. Mechanistically speaking, LDRT inhibits the production of pro-inflammatory cytokines like IL-6 and tumor necrosis factor-α (TNF-α) that are induced by the SARS-CoV-2 spike protein. Additionally, it counteracts the downregulation of angiotensin-converting enzyme 2 (ACE2) caused by the spike protein, restoring its normal physiological function [27]. Furthermore, LDRT promotes the generation of transforming growth factor-β (TGF-β), which facilitates the polarization or recruitment of M2 macrophages. This alteration reduces immune cell infiltration and moderates excessive inflammatory responses, thereby alleviating cytokine storm-like conditions [33]. Despite the potential benefits it offers, the application of LDRT in the treatment of COVID-19 has led to inconsistent results. Some research reveals that the mortality rate among COVID-19 patients remains high after LDRT [29, 34], while other studies suggest that LDRT has no significant impact on overall survival [35]. These differences highlight the variability in patient outcomes, which might potentially be influenced by factors such as patient demographics, disease severity, and study design. To establish the role of LDRT in COVID-19 management, larger-scale, rigorously designed randomized controlled trials are needed. Such studies should aim to identify optimal patient populations, dosage protocols, and timing of LDRT, as well as to assess its long-term effects and potential risks.

Radiological diagnosis has played an indispensable role in the early detection, assessment of disease progression, and monitoring of therapeutic outcomes in COVID-19. Diagnostic modalities such as chest X-rays, CT, and ultrasound provide timely and accurate insights into disease progression, serving as critical tools for guiding clinical decision-making. LDRT has demonstrated the capacity to alleviate symptoms and improve the quality of life for certain COVID-19 patients. However, the safety and efficacy of these methods require validation through large-scale, prospective clinical trials. Looking ahead, technological advancements and more in-depth exploration of radiological techniques will likely enhance their contributions to the prevention, diagnosis, and treatment of COVID-19 patients. These innovations will further strengthen the importance of radiology in safeguarding the health and well-being of patients during and even after the pandemic.

3. HBV virus

3.1 Introduction of HBV

Hepatitis B virus (HBV) infection is a significant global health concern, affecting approximately 350 million individuals worldwide [36]. Chronic HBV infection is a major risk factor for hepatocellular carcinoma (HCC), accounting for at least 50% of HCC cases globally [37]. Mechanisms Linking HBV to HCC include: (1) Direct integration and genomic instability: HBV can integrate its DNA into the host genome, leading to genomic instability and insertional mutagenesis of cancer-related genes [38]. (2) HBx protein: The HBV X protein (HBx) plays a central role in hepatocarcinogenesis by modulating various cellular pathways, including those involved in cell proliferation and apoptosis [39]. (3) Chronic inflammation: Persistent HBV infection leads to chronic liver inflammation, promoting a microenvironment conducive to carcinogenesis.

Radiotherapy (RT) has emerged as a pivotal treatment modality for HCC, especially in cases where surgical options are limited. However, HBV reactivation is a well-documented complication in patients undergoing chemotherapy, with reactivation rates ranging from 14% to 72% in hematological malignancies [40]. In the context of RT for HCC, HBV reactivation, though less frequently discussed, poses significant risks, including liver failure and mortality. A case study reported HBV reactivation leading to liver failure in a patient with HCC undergoing RT, despite prophylactic antiviral therapy with entecavir [41]. This underscores the necessity for vigilant monitoring and management of HBV DNA levels during RT to mitigate potential complications.

3.2 Advances in radiotherapy techniques for HBV-related HCC

The evolution of RT has introduced advanced modalities that enhance treatment precision and efficacy for HCC patients: External beam radiotherapy (EBRT): EBRT has transitioned from conventional techniques to sophisticated methods like intensity-modulated radiotherapy (IMRT) and stereotactic body radiotherapy (SBRT). These advancements have improved local tumor control and expanded the applicability of RT in HCC management [42]. Proton beam therapy (PBT): PBT offers superior dose distribution, minimizing radiation exposure to surrounding healthy tissues. This is particularly beneficial in HCC patients with compromised liver function due to chronic HBV infection. Studies have demonstrated the efficacy of PBT in achieving local control with reduced toxicity [42]. Given the risk of HBV reactivation during cancer treatment, guidelines recommend routine HBV screening for patients undergoing systemic chemotherapy [43]. While specific recommendations for RT are less established, the potential for HBV reactivation suggests that similar screening and prophylactic antiviral strategies should be considered for patients receiving RT, particularly those with known HBV infection. The intersection of HBV infection, HCC, and RT presents complex clinical challenges. Advancements in RT techniques have improved treatment outcomes for HBV-related HCC, yet the risk of HBV reactivation remains a critical concern. Comprehensive screening, vigilant monitoring, and the integration of antiviral prophylaxis are essential components of effective management strategies. Future research should continue to explore the optimization of RT modalities and the potential benefits of combining RT with immunotherapy to enhance therapeutic efficacy for HBV-related HCC patients.

4. HPV virus

4.1 Radiodiagnosis and radiotherapy of human papillomavirus-related cancers

Human papillomavirus (HPV), a common virus with over 200 types, infects skin and mucous membranes and is linked to various cancers. HPV types are divided into low-risk (e.g., types 6 and 11, causing genital warts) and high-risk (e.g., types 16 and 18, linked to cervical, anal, oropharyngeal, and penile cancers) [44]. HPV spreads through direct contact, and most sexually active individuals contract it, though many remain asymptomatic [45, 46]. However, HPV can lead to cancer over time, with E6 and E7 proteins causing cellular dysfunction and DNA damage [47, 48].

Radiological diagnostic techniques are vital for diagnosing and managing HPV-related cancers. Cervical cancer detection starts with cytology and HPV DNA tests, and imaging technologies like ultrasound, CT, MRI, and positron emission tomography (PET)-CT provide detailed tumor information for staging and treatment planning. Radiotherapy is a primary treatment for advanced cervical cancer, with imaging technologies crucial for accurate radiation targeting [49]. Advancements in radiological diagnostics and radiotherapy offer more precise tools for managing HPV-related cancers, improving treatment outcomes and patient survival rates [49, 50].

4.2 The role of imaging in diagnosing and managing HPV-related cervical cancer

Radiological imaging technologies play a multifaceted and essential role in the research and development of new therapies for HPV-related cancers. They provide a non-invasive method to assess the efficacy of new therapies, particularly in clinical trials. By comparing pre- and post-treatment imaging, researchers can quantify changes in tumor size, monitor tumor growth rates, and evaluate tumor responses to treatment. For example, in cervical cancer treatment, MRI can clearly show the relationship between the tumor and surrounding tissues, aiding in assessing tumor volume changes caused by radiotherapy or chemotherapy [50]. Moreover, radiological imaging technologies, especially PET-CT, offer insights into tumor metabolic activity, which is crucial for understanding tumor biology and predicting treatment responses. PET-CT, by measuring the glucose metabolism rate of tumor cells, can identify active tumor tissue, helping to distinguish residual active tumors from inactive fibrosis or necrotic tissue after treatment. In the development of new therapies, radiological imaging aids in early drug screening and dose determination. By monitoring tumor dynamics in experimental animal models, researchers can assess the anti-tumor activity of candidate drugs and set optimal drug doses for subsequent clinical trials. These technologies also support personalized medicine. Analyzing patients' imaging data allows doctors to craft precise treatment plans, such as selecting the most appropriate radiation therapy doses and targets or predicting responses to specific chemotherapy drugs. For monitoring disease progression, radiological imaging enables timely detection of tumor recurrence or metastasis, which is crucial for adjusting treatment strategies and improving patient prognosis. Regular CT scans, for instance, can track lung cancer patients' extrapulmonary metastasis, allowing for prompt treatment plan adjustments [51]. Overall, radiological imaging technologies are indispensable in the research and development of new therapies for HPV-related cancers. They help assess treatment outcomes, monitor disease progression, and advance the personalization and precision of cancer treatment, thereby enhancing treatment effectiveness, safety, and patient outcomes [49]. Radiological diagnosis is critical in managing HPV-related cancers. By employing imaging techniques such as ultrasound, CT, MRI, and PET-CT, doctors can accurately assess tumor size, shape, invasion extent, and distant metastasis. Advances in radiological diagnostic technologies have improved cancer detection rates and staging accuracy, providing patients with more effective treatment options [50, 52].

4.3 Radiotherapy in HPV-positive cervical cancer

4.3.1 How radiotherapy works in HPV-positive cervical cancer cells

Radiotherapy uses ionizing radiation to damage the DNA of cancer cells, either killing them or stopping their growth. In HPV-positive cervical cancer cells, the E6 and E7 proteins from the virus cause the loss of function of the tumor suppressor proteins p53 and Rb2. This makes the cells less able to repair DNA damage. When radiation causes breaks in the DNA, it triggers a response in the cell that usually stops the cell cycle to allow for DNA repair or to start cell death. However, in HPV-positive cells, the E6 protein speeds up the breakdown of p53, blocking this protective response, and the E7 protein binds to Rb, causing it to lose its function and allowing the cell cycle to go out of control [53, 54]. This damage to the repair process means that HPV-positive cells cannot fix DNA damage from radiotherapy as well as other cells, making them more likely to die. Additionally, different stages of the cell cycle react differently to radiotherapy. In HPV-positive cells, the loss of Rb function may make them more affected by radiotherapy during the S phase. Fractionated radiotherapy gives normal tissues time to repair damage between treatments, while cancer cells, with their weaker repair abilities, struggle to recover. This makes HPV-positive cervical cancer cells more sensitive to fractionated treatment. Radiotherapy can kill cancer cells through various methods, including apoptosis, necrosis, autophagy, or programmed necrosis. The inactivation of p53 and Rb in HPV-positive cells might affect how these methods are activated, making radiotherapy more effective. Overall, radiotherapy is more effective against HPV-positive cervical cancer cells because it directly damages DNA and affects cell cycle and cell death processes [54].

4.3.2 Radiotherapeutic sensitivity of different cell cycle phases

The sensitivity of radiotherapy varies among different phases of the cell cycle. Cells in the M phase and G1 phase are usually more resistant to radiotherapy because their DNA has already been copied or has not started copying yet, so damage may not lead to cell death. Cells in the S phase are more sensitive because DNA is being copied, and any damage could cause problems that lead to cell death. In HPV-positive cervical cancer cells, the E7 protein from the HPV virus binds to the Rb protein, causing it to lose its function and disrupting cell cycle control [55]. This makes cells unable to pause the cell cycle effectively when DNA damage is present, increasing the sensitivity of S-phase cells to radiotherapy. Normally, the Rb protein inhibits the E2F transcription factor, preventing cells from entering the S phase [56]. When Rb is inactive, E2F causes the expression of S phase-related genes to go out of control, pushing cells into the S phase and making them more affected by radiotherapy. Additionally, DNA damage from radiotherapy activates the DDR, and in S-phase cells, this can lead to unstable replication forks and an increased risk of DNA breaks, raising the chance of cell death. In contrast, cells in the M and G1 phases may have more chances to repair damage, making them more resistant to radiotherapy. In summary, HPV-positive cervical cancer cells have abnormal cell cycle control due to the loss of Rb function, making S-phase cells more sensitive to radiotherapy and providing a window for treatment. When planning radiotherapy, considering the cell cycle distribution and sensitivity of tumor cells can help improve treatment strategies and outcomes while reducing damage to normal tissues [57].

4.3.3 Dose-effect relationship of radiotherapy

The dose-effect relationship of radiotherapy is a key concept in radiation oncology, showing how radiotherapy dose relates to tumor control and normal tissue damage. In HPV-positive cervical cancer cells, the E6 and E7 proteins from the HPV virus interfere with the host cell's p53 and Rb proteins, leading to an uncontrolled cell cycle and impaired DNA repair [57]. This means HPV-positive cells are less able to fix DNA damage from radiotherapy, making them more sensitive to lower doses. This biological feature can change the shape of the dose-effect curve, making the tumor control probability curve steeper for HPV-positive tumors at lower doses, indicating that lower doses can achieve higher tumor control. Additionally, the increased sensitivity of HPV-positive cells may allow for lower radiotherapy doses without increasing the risk of normal tissue complications. This is important for protecting normal tissues, as they are generally less sensitive to radiotherapy than cancer tissues, but too high doses can still cause severe problems. In clinical practice, understanding this dose-effect relationship helps radiation oncologists optimize radiotherapy plans by adjusting doses and fractionation to achieve the best outcomes and minimal side effects. For HPV-positive cervical cancer patients, lower total doses and/or different fractionation patterns, like hyperfractionation, might be used to improve treatment and reduce damage to normal tissues. In summary, the increased sensitivity of HPV-positive cervical cancer cells to radiotherapy provides a window for effective treatment while protecting normal tissues [58]. This individualized approach requires considering the tumor's molecular characteristics, the patient's situation, and the technical capabilities of radiotherapy to achieve the best results.

4.3.4 Radiotherapy and HPV vaccines and screening

HPV vaccines are a major step forward in preventing cervical cancer, protecting against the most common HPV types that cause it, mainly HPV 16 and 18. However, vaccines cannot get rid of existing HPV infections or treat precancerous lesions or cancer that has already started. Therefore, regular screening and proper treatment are crucial for patients who have HPV, especially those with HPV-related cancers [44, 45]. Cervical cancer screening usually includes Pap smear tests and HPV DNA testing [59]. Using both methods together can increase the detection of precancerous lesions and cervical cancer. For patients with abnormal screening results, further tests like cervical biopsy or cervical conization may be needed to check for high-grade precancerous lesions or cancer. For treating HPV-related cancers, radiotherapy is a key method, especially when surgery is not possible or for mid-to-late-stage tumors. Radiotherapy uses ionizing radiation to damage the DNA of cancer cells, either killing them or stopping their growth. In HPV-positive cervical cancer cells, the loss of p53 and Rb protein function makes the cells less able to fix DNA damage, making them more sensitive to radiotherapy [60]. Radiotherapy is not only used for cervical cancer but also for other HPV-related cancers, like anal, oropharyngeal, and penile cancer. In these cases, radiotherapy can be the main treatment or used with chemotherapy to improve outcomes. It can also be used after surgery to lower the risk of recurrence. For cancers caused by HPV types not covered by the vaccine, radiotherapy is still important. Although these types of HPV infections are rare, they can still cause cancer. In these situations, the radiotherapy strategy and plan need to be tailored to the specific tumor and the patient's health. In summary, while HPV vaccines provide strong protection against HPV-related cancers, regular screening and proper treatment, including radiotherapy, are still key for managing patients who are already infected. Radiotherapy plays an essential role in the comprehensive treatment of HPV-related cancers [61], whether as the main treatment or combined with other methods, aiming to improve treatment outcomes and patient survival rates.

4.3.5 Long-term effects and side effect management of radiotherapy

The long-term effects and side effects management of radiotherapy are crucial for HPV-positive cervical cancer patients. After completing radiotherapy, long-term follow-up monitoring is essential to detect potential recurrences and metastases early [62]. This monitoring relies on radiological imaging techniques like CT, MRI, and PET-CT, which can provide detailed information about the tumor's behavior and spread without being invasive [52, 63–65]. Early detection of recurrence can lead to timely intervention and may improve survival and quality of life. Managing the side effects of radiotherapy is an important part of the treatment plan, especially for HPV-positive patients, who may be more sensitive to it. Short-term side effects can include skin inflammation, mucositis, and digestive system symptoms, while long-term side effects may include chronic pain, fibrosis, and organ dysfunction. To reduce these side effects, radiotherapy plans need to be individually adjusted to optimize dose distribution and protect surrounding normal tissues. For example, intensity modulated radiotherapy (IMRT) and image-guided radiotherapy (IGRT) can provide more precise dose control, reducing unnecessary exposure to normal tissues [66]. In the treatment plan, radiation oncologists consider the tumor's location, size, and extent of invasion, as well as the patient's individual differences, such as age, overall health, and coexisting conditions. Through precise dose calculation and treatment planning, the effectiveness of radiotherapy can be maximized while minimizing the risk of damage to normal tissues. Additionally, regular assessments during treatment and long-term follow-up after treatment, including symptom monitoring, quality of life evaluation, and necessary imaging tests, are important components of managing radiotherapy side effects [67]. In summary, for HPV-positive cervical cancer patients, long-term follow-up and side effect management after radiotherapy are key to ensuring the best treatment outcomes and patient quality of life. Through precise radiological monitoring and individualized radiotherapy plans, tumors can be effectively controlled while minimizing the long-term effects and side effects of radiotherapy.

5. Monkeypox virus

Monkeypox virus (MPXV) was first identified in monkeys, hence the name "monkeypox" [68]. It was first reported in humans in tropical regions of Central and

West Africa in 1970 [69]. The geographic spread of monkeypox and the number of reported cases outside Africa have increased since 2022, raising global public health concerns [68, 70]. MPXV is a double-stranded DNA virus belonging to the genus *Orthopoxvirus* of the *Poxviridae* family, which also includes variola and vaccinia viruses [71]. The virus has a typical brick-like or oval structure and is about 200–250 nanometers in diameter [72]. Its genome is approximately 200 kilobases long and encodes around 200 proteins that play important roles in virus production and the ability to infect host cells [73]. The MPXV genome consists of a highly conserved central core region, variable regions at both ends, and inverted terminal tandem repeats [72]. MPXV has two main clades: Clade I, which represents pre-Central African lineages, and Clade II, which represents West African lineages [74, 75]. Differences in genes encoding virulence between the two clades may be related to the varying severity of the disease they cause. Clade I is generally less pathogenic, while Clade II is associated with more severe clinical manifestations, including higher mortality [73].

5.1 Effect of immune response in patients with MPXV infection

MPXV enters the human body through mucous membranes and the skin, infecting immune cells and antigen-presenting cells in the tissues. It then spreads through the lymphatic system [76]. In the early stages of infection, monocytes recruited to the site of infection become early targets for the virus [77]. Although the number of natural killer (NK) cells in individuals infected with MPXV is increased, their immune function is significantly impaired [78]. Additionally, immune effector molecules play a crucial role during MPXV infection. At the onset of infection, the virus can inhibit the expression of chemokines, leading to reduced production of interferon-γ (IFN-γ), tumor necrosis factor-α (TNF-α), and other effector molecules [76]. This, in turn, affects T-cell activation and hinders the initiation of the humoral immune response, enabling the virus to evade the immune system more easily. Severe MPXV infection often leads to cytokine storms as the disease progresses. This results in an increase in T helper (Th)2-associated cytokines and a decrease in Th1-associated cytokines, characterized by elevated expression of IL-2, IL-4, and IL-8, and a reduction in TNF-α, IL-2, and IL-12 [78, 79]. Immunocompromised individuals are at a higher risk of developing severe disease and mortality when infected with the MPXV.

5.2 Potential molecular mechanisms of radiation therapy

MPXV first enters the body through the skin or mucous membranes and infects local immune cells and antigen-presenting cells such as monocytes and dendritic cells [80]. It can inhibit T cell activation by inhibiting the expression of chemokines, thereby inhibiting humoral immune responses and making it easier for the virus to evade immune surveillance [76]. Monkeypox viruses also regulate host cell signaling pathways and suppress immune responses by coding for specific proteins, such as Bcl-2 and SPI-2 proteins [81]. Bcl2-like proteins regulate apoptosis pathways, and SPI-2 proteins prevent pyro death or apoptosis by inhibiting caspase-1 and caspase-8, thereby avoiding the death of host cells and contributing to the long-term survival of viruses in host cells [82]. Radiotherapy induces DNA double-strand breaks through high-energy radiation, initiates DNA damage response (DDR), and activates key proteins such as ATM/ATR, p53, Chk1, and so on, thereby initiating cell cycle arrest, repair, or induce apoptosis, which may lead to the death of virus-infected cells and reduce virus spread [83]. Radiotherapy also activates dendritic cells, enhances the immune response of T cells, and enhances the killing of virus-infected cells by natural killer cells (NK cells) [84]. However, excessive cytokine release can lead to immune dysregulation, especially in the early stages of viral infection, potentially exacerbating immune damage.

6. Avian influenza virus

Avian influenza, commonly known as bird flu, is an infectious disease caused by an influenza virus that primarily affects birds [85]. The avian influenza virus (AIV) is an RNA virus from the genus *Influenza virus* of the family *Orthomyxoviridae*, with the influenza A subtype being most commonly associated with human infection. Based on two surface proteins—hemagglutinin (HA) and neuraminidase (NA)—these viruses are divided into different subtypes, resulting in various combinations such as H5N1, H7N9, and H9N2 [85, 86]. AIV belongs to the influenza A family of viruses. The viral genome consists of eight RNA segments that encode at least 10 proteins, including the surface glycoproteins hemagglutinin (HA) and neuraminidase (NA) [87]. These glycoproteins play a key role in the viral infection of host cells and viral transmission [86]. Avian influenza primarily affects wild waterfowl, such as ducks, geese, and swans, which act as natural reservoirs. These birds can carry the virus without showing symptoms. Domestic poultry (chickens, turkeys, ducks) can also be infected, often leading to severe outbreaks on farms, especially when the virus is highly pathogenic (such as H5N1 or H7N9) [88].

6.1 Effect of radiotherapy on immune response in patients with the viral infection

Radiation therapy (RT) is a common form of cancer treatment used to treat approximately 50% of cancer patients, either alone or in combination with other treatments, such as surgery, chemotherapy, immunotherapy, and targeted therapy [89]. Additionally, several studies have highlighted the potential of LDRT for the treatment of pneumonia [90]. Radiation therapy works by destroying cancer cells through direct DNA damage via ionization or indirectly by generating reactive oxygen species (ROS) [91]. Radiosensitivity is an inherent characteristic of tumor cells, which exhibit varying radiosensitivity at different stages of the cell cycle. The current fractionated radiotherapy regimen not only allows for the recovery of damaged normal cells, thereby reducing side effects but also reoxygenates tumor cells and redistributes them to more sensitive stages of the cell cycle, thereby increasing tumor damage [91]. Although radiation therapy can enhance the immunogenicity of tumors and alter the tumor microenvironment to promote immune destruction, circulating lymphocytes are also highly sensitive to radiation, leading to lymphocyte depletion. The reduction in lymphocytes is considered a factor contributing to the poor prognosis of many malignant tumors [92].

Influenza viruses are typically transmitted by inhaling aerosols containing virions, which enter through the mucous membranes of the respiratory tract. The innate immune system provides a strong barrier against influenza viruses. Viral RNA in infected cells is recognized by various pattern recognition receptors (PRRs), inducing the production of a variety of cytokines and chemokines [93]. Chemokines recruit immune cells, including mononuclear macrophages and neutrophils, to the site of infection and play an antiviral role. However, virus-induced cytokine dysregulation may exacerbate disease severity. The low T lymphocyte count and abnormally elevated chemokine and cytokine levels in the peripheral blood of H5N1-infected individuals are closely related to poor clinical prognosis [94].

6.2 Potential molecular mechanisms of radiation therapy

LDRT reduces interactions between white blood cells and endothelial cells by inhibiting nitric oxide synthase (iNOS), thereby reducing vasodilation and inflammatory responses [95]. Studies have shown that LDRT is able to promote the production of anti-inflammatory cytokines such as IL-10 and reduce leukocyte apoptosis and free radical formation by polarizing macrophages into M2 type, which helps mitigate tissue damage after influenza infection [96]. LDRT may also have a positive effect on viral pneumonia by reducing the inflammatory response in the lungs, especially by regulating the immune response, reducing the release of pro-inflammatory factors, and suppressing excessive immune responses [33]. LDRT may alleviate lung symptoms and acute respiratory distress syndrome (ARDS) by upregulating the expression of anti-inflammatory cytokines (such as IL-10) and inhibiting the expression of pro-inflammatory cytokines (such as IL-6 and IFN-γ), alleviating associated cytokine storms [33, 90]. In addition, LDRT may indirectly support antiviral therapy by activating immune response and enhancing antiviral response, which has potential therapeutic significance.

Radiation therapy, particularly low-dose ionizing radiation, has shown potential benefits in treating viral infections, including reducing inflammation and modulating immune responses. However, its effects on the immune system are complex, and the depletion of lymphocytes and potential immune dysregulation may worsen disease progression in viral infections like MPXV and AIV. Further research is needed to understand the dual role of RT in both enhancing immune responses and potentially exacerbating immune damage in patients with viral infections. Understanding these mechanisms could lead to more effective therapeutic strategies for managing viral infections, especially in immunocompromised patients.

7. Challenges and future directions

Despite the promising results, there are several challenges to overcome in the development of viral and radiation combination therapies. These include optimizing the timing and sequence of treatments, understanding the complex interactions between the virus, radiation, and the tumor microenvironment, and addressing potential side effects. The combination of viral infections and radiation therapy represents a novel and exciting frontier in cancer treatment. By harnessing the unique properties of oncolytic viruses and the established efficacy of radiation, this approach offers a multifaceted strategy to combat cancer. As research continues to advance, the integration of these therapies into clinical practice has the potential to significantly improve the prognosis for patients with various types of cancer.

8. Conclusion

In conclusion, the intricate interplay between viral infections and radiation therapy presents a multifaceted landscape with significant implications for both cancer treatment and the management of viral diseases. This chapter has explored the complex relationships between various viruses and radiation, highlighting the potential benefits and challenges of combining these modalities. For specific viral infections such as COVID-19, HBV, HPV, monkeypox, and avian influenza, radiation therapy has shown potential in modulating the immune response and reducing inflammation. The combination of viral therapies and radiation presents a promising frontier in cancer treatment and viral disease management. As research continues to advance, the optimization of treatment protocols, the development of personalized medicine approaches, and the integration of immunotherapy will be crucial for realizing the full potential of these combined therapies. Future directions should focus on overcoming the challenges of treatment optimization, understanding complex interactions, and addressing potential side effects to improve patient outcomes.

Abbreviations

ACE2	angiotensin-converting enzyme 2
AIV	avian influenza virus
ARDS	acute respiratory distress syndrome
ATM	Ataxia telangiectasia mutated proteins
ATR	Ataxia telangiectasia and Rad3-related protein
Bcl-2	B-cell lymphoma-2
Chk1	checkpoint kinase 1
COVID-19	coronavirus disease 2019
CRP	C-reactive protein
CT	computed tomography
DDR	DNA damage response
DWI	diffusion-weighted imaging
EBRT	external beam radiotherapy
E2F	early 2 factor
GGOs	ground-glass opacities
HA	hemagglutinin
HBV	hepatitis B virus
HBx	HBV X protein
HCC	hepatocellular carcinoma
HPV	human papillomavirus
HRCT	high-resolution computed tomography
IFN-γ	interferon-γ
IGRT	image-guided radiotherapy
IL-6	interleukin-6
IMRT	intensity-modulated radiotherapy
iNOS	inhibiting nitric oxide synthase
LDH	lactate dehydrogenase
LDRT	low-dose ionizing radiation therapy
LDRT	low-dose radiotherapy
MPXV	monkeypox virus
MRI	magnetic resonance imaging
NA	neuraminidase
NK	natural killer
NK cells	natural killer cells

PBT	proton beam therapy
PET-CT	positron emission tomography-computed tomography
PRRs	pattern recognition receptors
p53	protein 53
Rb	retinoblastoma
ROS	reactive oxygen species
RT	radiotherapy
SARS-CoV-2	severe acute respiratory syndrome coronavirus-2
SBRT	stereotactic body radiotherapy
SPI-2	salmonella pathogenicity island-2
TGF-β	transforming growth factor-β
TNF-α	tumor necrosis factor-α

Author details

Yu Zhao[1*†], Yingyi Zhang[2†], Yang Liu[1†], Junling Zhang[1†], Sen Wang[1†], Danyue Qu[1], Xinyuan Ji[1] and Saijun Fan[1*]

1 Tianjin Key Laboratory of Radiation Medicine and Molecular Nuclear Medicine, Institute of Radiation Medicine, Chinese Academy of Medical Sciences and Peking Union Medical College, Tianjin, P.R. China

2 School of Disaster and Emergency Medicine, Tianjin University, Tianjin, P.R. China

*Address all correspondence to: zhaoyu@irm-cams.ac.cn
and fansaijun@irm-cams.ac.cn

† These authors contributed equally.

References

[1] Magon KL, Parish JL. From infection to cancer: How DNA tumour viruses alter host cell central carbon and lipid metabolism. Open Biology. 2021;**11**(3):210004

[2] McAllister RM. Viruses and cancer. California Medicine. 1965;**102**(5):344-352

[3] Tashiro H, Brenner MK. Immunotherapy against cancer-related viruses. Cell Research. 2017;**27**(1):59-73

[4] Studstill CJ, Mac M, Moody CA. Interplay between the DNA damage response and the life cycle of DNA tumor viruses. Tumour Virus Research. 2023;**16**:200272

[5] Hemminki O, Dos Santos JM, Hemminki A. Oncolytic viruses for cancer immunotherapy. Journal of Hematology & Oncology. 2020;**13**(1):84

[6] Bommareddy PK, Shettigar M, Kaufman HL. Integrating oncolytic viruses in combination cancer immunotherapy. Nature Reviews. Immunology. 2018;**18**(8):498-513

[7] Zou X, Ren Y, Yang H, Zou M, Meng P, Zhang L, et al. Screening and staging of chronic obstructive pulmonary disease with deep learning based on chest X-ray images and clinical parameters. BMC Pulmonary Medicine. 2024;**24**(1):153

[8] Yamasaki Y, Hosokawa K, Abe K, Ishigami K. Dynamic chest radiography of acute pulmonary thromboembolism. Radiology: Cardiothoracic Imaging. 2022;**4**(4):e220086

[9] Pal A, Ali A, Young TR, Oostenbrink J, Prabhakar A, Prabhakar A, et al. Comprehensive literature review on the radiographic findings, imaging modalities, and the role of radiology in the COVID-19 pandemic. World Journal of Radiology. 2021;**13**(9):258-282

[10] Martínez Chamorro E, Díez Tascón A, Ibáñez Sanz L, Ossaba Vélez S, Borruel Nacenta S. Radiologic diagnosis of patients with COVID-19. Radiología (English Edition). 2021;**63**(1):56-73

[11] Aljondi R, Alghamdi S. Diagnostic value of imaging modalities for COVID-19: Scoping review. Journal of Medical Internet Research. 2020;**22**(8):e19673

[12] Sofia S, Orlandi P, Bua V, Imbriani M, Cecilioni L, Caruso A, et al. Lung ultrasound and high-resolution computed tomography in suspected COVID-19 patients admitted to the emergency department: A comparison. Journal of Diagnostic Medical Sonography. 2023;**39**(4):332-346

[13] Abedi I, Vali M, Otroshi B, Zamanian M, Bolhasani H. HRCTCov19-a high-resolution chest CT scan image dataset for COVID-19 diagnosis and differentiation. BMC Research Notes. 2024;**17**(1):32

[14] Al-Momani H. A literature review on the relative diagnostic accuracy of chest CT scans versus RT-PCR testing for COVID-19 diagnosis. Tomography. 2024;**10**(6):935-948

[15] Sanli DET, Yildirim D, Sanli AN, Turkmen S, Erozan N, Husmen G, et al. A practical approach to imaging characteristics and standardized reporting of COVID-19: A radiologic review. Military Medical Research. 2021;**8**(1):7

[16] Mira JG, Potter JL, Fullerton GD, Ezekiel J. Advantages and limitations

of computed tomography scans for treatment planning of lung cancer. International Journal of Radiation Oncology, Biology, Physics. 1982;**8**(9):1617-1623

[17] Cellina M, Martinenghi C, Marino P, Oliva G. COVID-19 pneumonia-ultrasound, radiographic, and computed tomography findings: A comprehensive pictorial essay. Emergency Radiology. 2021;**28**(3):519-526

[18] Allinovi M, Parise A, Giacalone M, Amerio A, Delsante M, Odone A, et al. Lung ultrasound may support diagnosis and monitoring of COVID-19 pneumonia. Ultrasound in Medicine & Biology. 2020;**46**(11):2908-2917

[19] Zaki HA, Albaroudi B, Shaban EE, Shaban A, Elgassim M, Almarri ND, et al. Advancement in pleura effusion diagnosis: A systematic review and meta-analysis of point-of-care ultrasound versus radiographic thoracic imaging. Ultrasound Journal. 2024;**16**(1):3

[20] Grimberg A, Shigueoka DC, Atallah AN, Ajzen S, Iared W. Diagnostic accuracy of sonography for pleural effusion: Systematic review. São Paulo Medical Journal. 2010;**128**(2):90-95

[21] Syrjala H, Broas M, Ohtonen P, Jartti A, Pääkkö E. Chest magnetic resonance imaging for pneumonia diagnosis in outpatients with lower respiratory tract infection. The European Respiratory Journal. 2017;**49**(1):1601303

[22] Konietzke P, Mueller J, Wuennemann F, Wagner WL, Schenk JP, Alrajab A, et al. The value of chest magnetic resonance imaging compared to chest radiographs with and without additional lung ultrasound in children with complicated pneumonia. PLoS ONE. 2020;**15**(3):e0230252

[23] Yang S, Zhang Y, Shen J, Dai Y, Ling Y, Lu H, et al. Clinical potential of UTE-MRI for assessing COVID-19: Patient- and lesion-based comparative analysis. Journal of Magnetic Resonance Imaging. 2020;**52**(2):397-406

[24] Torkian P, Rajebi H, Zamani T, Ramezani N, Kiani P, Akhlaghpoor S. Magnetic resonance imaging features of coronavirus disease 2019 (COVID-19) pneumonia: The first preliminary case series. Clinical Imaging;**69**(2021):261-265

[25] Chalkia M, Arkoudis NA, Maragkoudakis E, Rallis S, Tremi I, Georgakilas AG, et al. The role of ionizing radiation for diagnosis and treatment against COVID-19: Evidence and considerations. Cells. 2022;**11**(3):467

[26] Pandey SR, Adhikari Yadav S, Gautam S, Giri K, Devkota A, Shrestha S, et al. Effectiveness of low-dose radiation therapy in COVID-19 patients globally: A systematic review. F1000Res. 2022;**11**:62

[27] Wen K, Bai C, Zhao H, Zhou P, Gao S, Guan H, et al. Low dose radiation therapy attenuates ACE2 depression and inflammatory cytokines induction by COVID-19 viral spike protein in human bronchial epithelial cells. International Journal of Radiation Biology. 2022;**98**(10):1532-1541

[28] Sanmamed N, Alcantara P, Gómez S, Bustos A, Cerezo E, Gaztañaga M, et al. Low-dose radiation therapy in the management of COVID-19 pneumonia (LOWRAD-Cov19). Final results of a prospective phase I-II trial. Radiotherapy and Oncology. 2022;**171**:25-29

[29] Arenas M, Piqué B, Torres-Royo L, Acosta JC, Rodríguez-Tomàs E, De Febrer G, et al. Treatment of COVID-19 pneumonia with low-dose radiotherapy plus standard of care versus standard of care alone in frail patients: The

SEOR-GICOR IPACOVID comparative cohort trial. Strahlentherapie und Onkologie. 2023;**199**(9):847-856

[30] Rutkowski TW, Jaroszewicz J, Piotrowski D, Ślosarek K, Sobala-Szczygieł B, Słonina D, et al. Low-dose radiotherapy for patients with pneumonia due to COVID-19: A single-institution prospective study. Biomedicine. 2023;**11**(3):858

[31] Rodríguez-Tomàs E, Acosta JC, Torres-Royo L, De Febrer G, Baiges-Gaya G, Castañé H, et al. Effect of low-dose radiotherapy on the circulating levels of paraoxonase-1-related variables and markers of inflammation in patients with COVID-19 pneumonia. Antioxidants (Basel). 2022;**11**(6):1184

[32] Dinakar K, Jakka MK, Vemannagari PKR, Mohan A, Subramanian BV, Bodagala VD, et al. Efficacy of low-dose lung radiotherapy in the management of COVID-19 patients: A randomised, open-label study. The British Journal of Radiology. 2023;**96**(1152):20230022

[33] Song HY, Chen F, Park HR, Han JM, Ji HJ, Byun EB, et al. Low-dose radiation therapy suppresses viral pneumonia by enhancing broad-spectrum anti-inflammatory responses via transforming growth factor-β production. Frontiers in Immunology. 2023;**14**:1182927

[34] Magrini SM, Tomasini D, Focà E, Garrafa EM, Singh N, Guerini AE, et al. Low-dose lung radiotherapy for COVID-19-related pneumonia: Preliminary results of the Italian mono-institutional COLOR-19 trial. In Vivo. 2022;**36**(4):1959-1965

[35] Kolahdouzan K, Chavoshi M, Bayani R, Darzikolaee NM. Low-dose whole lung irradiation for treatment of COVID-19 pneumonia: A systematic review and meta-analysis. International Journal of Radiation Oncology, Biology, Physics. 2022;**113**(5):946-959

[36] Hsu YC, Huang DQ, Nguyen MH. Global burden of hepatitis B virus: Current status, missed opportunities and a call for action. Nature Reviews. Gastroenterology & Hepatology. 2023;**20**(8):524-537

[37] Xie Y. Hepatitis B virus-associated hepatocellular carcinoma. Advances in Experimental Medicine and Biology. 2017;**1018**:11-21

[38] Levrero M, Zucman-Rossi J. Mechanisms of HBV-induced hepatocellular carcinoma. Journal of Hepatology. 2016;**64**(Suppl. 1):S84-S101

[39] Rizzo GEM, Cabibbo G, Craxi A. Hepatitis B virus-associated hepatocellular carcinoma. Viruses. 2022;**14**(5)

[40] Voican CS, Mir O, Loulergue P, Dhooge M, Brezault C, Dreanic J, et al. Hepatitis B virus reactivation in patients with solid tumors receiving systemic anticancer treatment. Annals of Oncology: Official Journal of the European Society for Medical Oncology. 2016;**27**(12):2172-2184

[41] Cheng J, Pei HH, Sun J, Xie QX, Li JB. Radiation-induced hepatitis B virus reactivation in hepatocellular carcinoma: A case report. Oncology Letters. 2015;**10**(5):3213-3215

[42] Kim D, Kim JS. Current perspectives on radiotherapy in hepatocellular carcinoma management: A comprehensive review. Journal of Liver Cancer. 2024;**24**(1):33-46

[43] Hwang JP, Feld JJ, Hammond SP, Wang SH, Alston-Johnson DE, Cryer DR, et al. Hepatitis B virus screening and

management for patients with cancer prior to therapy: ASCO provisional clinical opinion update. Journal of Clinical Oncology: Official Journal of the American Society of Clinical Oncology. 2020;**38**(31):3698-3715

[44] Bosch FX, Lorincz A, Munoz N, Meijer CJ, Shah KV. The causal relation between human papillomavirus and cervical cancer. Journal of Clinical Pathology. 2002;**55**(4):244-265

[45] de Martel C, Georges D, Bray F, Ferlay J, Clifford GM. Global burden of cancer attributable to infections in 2018: A worldwide incidence analysis. The Lancet Global Health. 2020;**8**(2):e180-e190

[46] Mahdi AGM. Knowledge, and attitude of medical students about role of human papilloma virus, and vaccine in head and neck cancer. Oral Oncology. 2024;**156**:106939

[47] Chong JS, Doorbar J. Modulation of epithelial homeostasis by HPV using notch and Wnt. Tumour Virus Research. 2024;**18**:200297

[48] Manini I, Montomoli E. Epidemiology and prevention of human papillomavirus. Annali di Igiene. 2018;**30**(4 Supple. 1):28-32

[49] Salzillo TC, Taku N, Wahid KA, McDonald BA, Wang J, van Dijk LV, et al. Advances in imaging for HPV-related oropharyngeal cancer: Applications to radiation oncology. Seminars in Radiation Oncology. 2021;**31**(4):371-388

[50] Krishnamurthy A, Ramshankar V. Current status and future perspectives of molecular prevention strategies for cervical cancers. Indian Journal of Surgical Oncology. 2020;**11**(4):752-761

[51] Rahaman A, Anantharaju A, Jeyachandran K, Manideep R, Pal UM. Optical imaging for early detection of cervical cancer: State of the art and perspectives. Journal of Biomedical Optics. 2023;**28**(8):080902

[52] Jo KH, Kim J, Cho H, Kang WJ, Lee SK, Sohn B. (18)F-FDG PET/CT parameters enhance MRI radiomics for predicting human papilloma virus status in oropharyngeal squamous cell carcinoma. Yonsei Medical Journal. 2023;**64**(12):738-744

[53] World Health Organization. Human papillomavirus vaccines: WHO position paper, May 2017. Weekly Epidemiological Record. 2017;**92**(19):241-268

[54] Doorbar J, Quint W, Banks L, Bravo IG, Stoler M, Broker TR, et al. The biology and life-cycle of human papillomaviruses. Vaccine. 2012;**30**(Suppl. 5):F55-F70

[55] Yim EK, Park JS. The role of HPV E6 and E7 oncoproteins in HPV-associated cervical carcinogenesis. Cancer Research and Treatment. 2005;**37**(6):319-324

[56] Idres YM, McMillan NAJ, Idris A. Hyperactivating p53 in human papillomavirus-driven cancers: A potential therapeutic intervention. Molecular Diagnosis & Therapy. 2022;**26**(3):301-308

[57] Pal A, Kundu R. Human papillomavirus E6 and E7: The cervical cancer hallmarks and targets for therapy. Frontiers in Microbiology. 2019;**10**:3116

[58] Huang Y, Zou D, Guo M, He M, He H, Li X, et al. HPV and radiosensitivity of cervical cancer: A narrative review. Annals of Translational Medicine. 2022;**10**(24):1405

[59] Gandullia E, Bonioli E, Monteverde R, La Fauci MF, Lattere M, Augeri C, et al. Significance of the

evaluation of C-peptide in children with type 1 diabetes mellitus. La Pediatria Medica e Chirurgica. 1986;**8**(5):687-689

[60] Moody CA, Laimins LA. Human papillomavirus oncoproteins: Pathways to transformation. Nature Reviews. Cancer. 2010;**10**(8):550-560

[61] Someya M, Fukushima Y, Hasegawa T, Tsuchiya T, Kitagawa M, Gocho T, et al. Radiotherapy for HPV-related cancers: Prediction of therapeutic effects based on the mechanism of tumor immunity and the application of immunoradiotherapy. Japanese Journal of Radiology. 2022;**40**(5):458-465

[62] Cheng L, Wang Y, Du J. Human papillomavirus vaccines: An updated review. Vaccines (Basel). 2020;**8**(3)

[63] Pouyiourou M, Regnery S, Bochtler T, Herfarth K, Kramer A. Cancer of unknown primary (CUP)-single-site, oligometastatic, and in the head and neck region. Radiologie (Heidelberg, Germany). 2023;**63**(5):358-365

[64] Grigsby PW. The prognostic value of PET and PET/CT in cervical cancer. Cancer Imaging. 2008;**8**(1):146-155

[65] Morey T, Hodge JC, Stern C, Krishnan S, Foreman A. Correlation between radiologic and pathologic extranodal extension in HPV-associated oropharyngeal cancer: Systematic review. Head & Neck. 2022;**44**(12):2875-2885

[66] Rios I, Vasquez I, Cuervo E, Garzon O, Burbano J. Problems and solutions in IGRT for cervical cancer. Reports of Practical Oncology and Radiotherapy. 2018;**23**(6):517-527

[67] Yao Q, Wang J, Elfstrom KM, Strander B, Dillner J, Sundstrom K. Evaluation of primary HPV-based cervical screening among older women: Long-term follow-up of a randomized healthcare policy trial in Sweden. PLoS Medicine. 2024;**21**(12):e1004505

[68] Harapan H, Ophinni Y, Megawati D, Frediansyah A, Mamada SS, Salampe M, et al. Monkeypox: A comprehensive review. Viruses. 2022;**14**(10)

[69] Ladnyj ID, Ziegler P, Kima E. A human infection caused by monkeypox virus in Basankusu Territory, Democratic Republic of the Congo. Bulletin of the World Health Organization. 1972;**46**(5):593-597

[70] Elsayed S, Bondy L, Hanage WP. Monkeypox virus infections in humans. Clinical Microbiology Reviews. 2022;**35**(4):e0009222

[71] Yi XM, Lei YL, Li M, Zhong L, Li S. The monkeypox virus-host interplays. Cell Insight. 2024;**3**(5):100185

[72] Huang Y, Mu L, Wang W. Monkeypox: Epidemiology, pathogenesis, treatment and prevention. Signal Transduction and Targeted Therapy. 2022;**7**(1):373

[73] Mitjà O, Ogoina D, Titanji BK, Galvan C, Muyembe JJ, Marks M, et al. Monkeypox. Lancet (London, England). 2023;**401**(10370):60-74

[74] Cevik M, Tomori O, Mbala P, Scagliarini A, Petersen E, Low N, et al. The 2023-2024 multi-source mpox outbreaks of Clade I MPXV in sub-Saharan Africa: Alarm bell for Africa and the World. International Journal of Infectious Diseases: IJID: Official Publication of the International Society for Infectious Diseases. 2024;**146**:107159

[75] Forni D, Molteni C, Cagliani R, Sironi M. Geographic structuring and divergence time frame of Monkeypox

virus in the endemic region. The Journal of Infectious Diseases. 2023;**227**(6):742-751

[76] Lu J, Xing H, Wang C, Tang M, Wu C, Ye F, et al. Mpox (formerly monkeypox): Pathogenesis, prevention, and treatment. Signal Transduction and Targeted Therapy. 2023;**8**(1):458

[77] Nikitina E, Larionova I, ChoinzonovE,KzhyshkowskaJ.Monocytes and macrophages as viral targets and reservoirs. International Journal of Molecular Sciences. 2018;**19**(9)

[78] Li H, Huang QZ, Zhang H, Liu ZX, Chen XH, Ye LL, et al. The land-scape of immune response to monkeypox virus. eBioMedicine. 2023;**87**:104424

[79] Chan PK. Outbreak of avian influenza A(H5N1) virus infection in Hong Kong in 1997. Clinical Infectious Diseases : An Official Publication of the Infectious Diseases Society of America. 2002;**34**(Suppl. 2):S58-S64

[80] El Eid R, Allaw F, Haddad SF, Kanj SS. Human monkeypox: A review of the literature. PLoS Pathogens. 2022;**18**(9):e1010768

[81] Lucena-Neto FD, Falcão LFM, Vieira-Junior AS, Moraes ECS, David JPF, Silva CC, et al. Monkeypox virus immune evasion and eye manifestation: Beyond eyelid implications. Viruses. 2023;**15**(12):2301

[82] Kvansakul M, Caria S, Hinds MG. The Bcl-2 family in host-virus interactions. Viruses. 2017;**9**(10):290

[83] García MEG, Kirsch DG, Reitman ZJ. Targeting the ATM kinase to enhance the efficacy of radiotherapy and outcomes for cancer patients. Seminars in Radiation Oncology. 2022;**32**(1):3-14

[84] McMahon RA, D'Souza C, Neeson PJ, Siva S. Innate immunity: Looking beyond T-cells in radiation and immunotherapy combinations. Neoplasia (New York, N.Y.). 2023;**46**:100940

[85] Zhu W, Yang L, Han X, Tan M, Zou S, Li X, et al. Origin, pathogenicity, and transmissibility of a human isolated influenza A(H10N3) virus from China. Emerging Microbes & Infections. 2025;**14**(1):2432364

[86] Charostad J, Rukerd MRZ, Mahmoudvand S, Bashash D, Hashemi SMA, Nakhaie M, et al. A comprehensive review of highly pathogenic avian influenza (HPAI) H5N1: An imminent threat at doorstep. Travel Medicine and Infectious Disease. 2023;**55**:102638

[87] Bouvier NM, Palese P. The biology of influenza viruses. Vaccine. 2008;**26**(Suppl. 4):D49-D53

[88] Bao P, Liu Y, Zhang X, Fan H, Zhao J, Mu M, et al. Human infection with a reassortment avian influenza A H3N8 virus: An epidemiological investigation study. Nature Communications. 2022;**13**(1):6817

[89] Olivares-Urbano MA, Griñán-Lisón C, Marchal JA, Núñez MI. CSC radioresistance: A therapeutic challenge to improve radiotherapy effectiveness in cancer. Cells. 2020;**9**(7):1651

[90] García-Hernández T, Romero-Expósito M, Sánchez-Nieto B. Low dose radiation therapy for COVID-19: Effective dose and estimation of cancer risk. Radiotherapy and Oncology: Journal of the European Society for Therapeutic Radiology and Oncology. 2020;**153**:289-295

[91] Lee SY, Jeong EK, Ju MK, Jeon HM, Kim MY, Kim CH, et al. Induction of

metastasis, cancer stem cell phenotype, and oncogenic metabolism in cancer cells by ionizing radiation. Molecular Cancer. 2017;**16**(1):10

[92] Zhao J, Huang W, Wu Y, Luo Y, Wu B, Cheng J, et al. Prognostic role of pretreatment blood lymphocyte count in patients with solid tumors: A systematic review and meta-analysis. Cancer Cell International. 2020;**20**:15

[93] Iwasaki A, Pillai PS. Innate immunity to influenza virus infection. Nature Reviews. Immunology. 2014;**14**(5):315-328

[94] Xie Y, Yu Y, Zhao L, Ning P, Luo Q, Zhang Y, et al. Specific cytokine profiles predict the severity of influenza A pneumonia: A prospectively multicenter pilot study. BioMed Research International. 2021;**2021**:9533044

[95] Tran N, Garcia T, Aniqa M, Ali S, Ally A, Nauli SM. Endothelial nitric oxide synthase (eNOS) and the cardiovascular system: In physiology and in disease states. American Journal of Biomedical Science and Research. 2022;**15**(2):153-177

[96] Boehler RM, Kuo R, Shin S, Goodman AG, Pilecki MA, Gower RM, et al. Lentivirus delivery of IL-10 to promote and sustain macrophage polarization towards an anti-inflammatory phenotype. Biotechnology and Bioengineering. 2014;**111**(6):1210-1221

Section 4

Novel Approaches to Treat Infectious Viral Diseases and Predict Host-Viral Interactions

Chapter 7

Wolbachia: From Natural Variation to Genetic Engineering – Exploring Gene-Level Approaches for Next-Generation Dengue Control

Iqra Mushtaq, Ammara Chaudhry and Muhammad Sajjad Sarwar

Abstract

Dengue fever poses a significant global health challenge, particularly in tropical and subtropical regions. Current control strategies, heavily reliant on vector control, face limitations due to insecticide resistance and logistical challenges in large urban areas. This book chapter explores the innovative potential of *Wolbachia* bacteria as a biocontrol agent against dengue. *Wolbachia* infection in *Aedes aegypti* mosquitoes, the primary dengue vector, has demonstrated promising results in reducing both viral replication within the mosquito and onward transmission to humans. This chapter examines the complex mechanisms underlying *Wolbachia*'s antiviral effects, including both immune system modulation and competition for host cell resources. Furthermore, the role of gene expression changes in mediating these effects, highlighting the potential for long-term, sustainable dengue suppression, is discussed. While challenges remain in large-scale implementation and the potential for viral evolution, *Wolbachia*-based interventions offer a new avenue for integrated vector management and hold considerable promise for reducing the global burden of dengue fever. Gene drive technology and thorough testing, such as analyzing virus sequences, are also discussed to evaluate how well *Wolbachia* works.

Keywords: *Wolbachia*, dengue virus, *Aedes aegypti*, viral inhibition, vector control

1. Introduction

Dengue fever, a viral disease spread by mosquitoes, is common in warm climates. Many people do not experience symptoms, but others may have a fever, headache, body pain, nausea, and rash. Recovery usually takes 1–2 weeks. Severe dengue requires hospitalization and can be fatal. Dengue fever has seen a dramatic rise globally in recent decades. The year 2023 saw the highest number of dengue cases on record, impacting over 80 countries across all WHO regions [1]. A significant increase in cases recently led to over 6.5 million reported cases and more than 7300 deaths, representing a record high. Global health authorities suggest that the majority

IntechOpen

of those affected live in the Asia-Pacific area. Several issues likely play a role in the region's high numbers, such as challenges in controlling the mosquito population, limited access to vaccines, less-than-ideal medical care, and weaknesses in public health systems [2]. South Asian countries, including those in the Indian subcontinent, are particularly vulnerable.

There is an increasing public health need for effective dengue prevention. Currently, two vaccines are licensed: Dengvaxia® (CYD-TDV) by Sanofi Pasteur and Qdenga® (TAK-003) by Takeda. Additionally, a third vaccine, developed by the National Institutes of Allergy and Infectious Diseases (NIAID), is in late-stage clinical trials [3]. But still, efforts to stop dengue depend greatly on controlling the *Aedes aegypti* mosquito, the main carrier. Unfortunately, these control efforts have not been very successful, mostly because they have not received enough funding and because it is hard to implement them effectively in large, densely populated areas and major cities [4]. Traditional methods for controlling dengue-carrying mosquitoes are often slow and ineffective [5]. The effectiveness of chemical control is severely compromised by widespread insecticide resistance in areas where dengue is common [6]. Additionally, global warming is causing the geographic range of *Ae. aegypti* and *Ae. albopictus* mosquitoes to expand northward. Once confined to tropical and subtropical zones, these mosquitoes are now spreading to temperate regions, including parts of Europe and North America [7]. Studies have shown that fluctuating temperatures can specifically impact dengue virus infection rates and transmission potential in mosquitoes. In response to these challenges, researchers are exploring the use of *Wolbachia* bacteria to reduce mosquito-borne virus transmission, including dengue. While some variability has been observed, *Wolbachia* has consistently reduced dengue infection and spread in several locations, notably Cairns, Australia, across a range of temperatures. This suggests that in suitable environments, *Wolbachia* could be a reliable tool for the biological control of dengue [8].

Wolbachia pipientis, an endosymbiotic bacterium first discovered in *Culex* mosquitoes in the 1920s [9], infects an estimated two-thirds of all insect species [10]. Its evolutionary success is attributed to its diverse manipulation of host biology. This maternally inherited endosymbiont strongly influences host characteristics, including reproduction [11], fitness [12, 13], metabolism [14], immunity [15, 16], and native microbiome [17, 18]. Current *Wolbachia*-based mosquito control programs primarily utilize cytoplasmic incompatibility (CI) [19] and pathogen blocking [20]. *Wolbachia*-induced CI was initially proposed for *Culex* mosquito control in 1967 [21]. CI boosts the number of *Wolbachia*-infected individuals in a population. Females with *Wolbachia* can reproduce normally with males that lack the infection or carry the same or a compatible strain of the bacteria [22]. CI happens when a male with a *Wolbachia* infection mates with a female that either does not have the same infection or has a different, incompatible strain [11]. In essence, incompatibility occurs when the male's *Wolbachia* strain differs from the female's.

Wolbachia impacts viruses by reducing or delaying viral accumulation and decreasing or delaying virus-induced mosquito mortality. While vector competence for arbovirus transmission is complex, *Wolbachia* can alter it by affecting mosquito susceptibility to viral infection [23–25]. Following its discovery in *Culex pipiens*, this endosymbiont has been found naturally in various mosquito species. Research indicates natural *Wolbachia* presence in varying proportions across mosquito genera: 7–42% in *Culex*, 0–30% in *Aedes*, and 1–15% in *Anopheles* [26–28]. Notably, *Wolbachia* is commonly found in important arbovirus vectors like the *Cx. pipiens* complex and *Aedes* species (including *Ae. albopictus*), but not *Ae. aegypti*. The native microbiome can impede *Wolbachia* establishment in some species, potentially explaining its absence [29]. However, artificial horizontal transfer of *Wolbachia* strains into both uninfected and already-infected hosts has been successfully demonstrated [30].

Modern biotechnology tools applied to area-wide integrated pest management are being used to develop both self-sustaining and self-limiting approaches. Self-sustaining strategies utilize population replacement with *Wolbachia*-based pathogen blocking, while self-limiting strategies employ population suppression via the *Wolbachia*-based incompatible insect technique [31, 32]. Due to insecticide resistance and the lack of effective vaccines, *Wolbachia* has been extensively studied as a novel mosquito vector control method. Over the last decade, *Wolbachia*-based strategies have progressed from small-scale field trials to larger efforts aimed at community-wide disease reduction. These advancements have led the WHO to recommend *Wolbachia*-based interventions for global dengue elimination in 2022 [33]. This chapter summarizes current knowledge of DENV control strategies, focusing on dengue elimination through *Wolbachia* interventions. It also discusses recent progress in *Wolbachia*-based control of dengue vectors.

2. How does the environment fuel dengue?

In dengue-endemic areas, environmental factors such as standing water, poor housing, and lack of air conditioning increase the abundance and distribution of *Ae. aegypti* and other *Aedes* spp. mosquitoes. These factors, along with climatic conditions like temperature, precipitation, and humidity, contribute to an increased risk of dengue transmission [34–36]. It is expected that climate change will worsen the dengue risk, mainly by intensifying transmission in areas where the disease already exists, and to a lesser extent by expanding the geographical distribution of *Aedes* mosquitoes [36, 37]. The increasing prevalence of dengue fever worldwide is influenced by more than just mosquitoes and climate. The development of cities, with their dense populations, provides ideal conditions for the disease to spread easily. The movement of people and the increasing challenges of poverty and displacement also contribute to the rise in cases since those in vulnerable situations often live in areas with poor sanitation and limited access to medical care, which increases their risk of infection. These linked social and environmental elements are predicted to substantially increase the global impact of dengue [38–41].

Travel plays a significant role in dengue's spread, carrying the virus to new areas where mosquitoes can transmit it or introducing different dengue types to places where it already exists [39, 42]. The introduction of new serotypes increases the risk for antibody-dependent enhancement and severe disease [43, 44]. Climate change is also a major factor in the spread and resurgence of mosquito-borne diseases worldwide [45]. Rising temperatures, changing rainfall, and more frequent extreme weather events are significantly altering where mosquitoes live, how many there are, and how quickly they reproduce. Rising temperatures accelerate mosquito spread, shorten the time it takes for viruses to develop within mosquitoes, and lengthen the disease transmission season, especially in areas previously too cold for mosquitoes to survive. Changes in rainfall also impact mosquito breeding sites; both too much and too little rain can create ideal conditions for mosquito breeding. As a result, dengue and other arboviruses are spreading to new areas, emphasizing the growing need for better surveillance and control [46]. The combined impact of environmental factors like climate change, alongside social factors such as urbanization, poverty, and migration, will likely intensify the dengue threat for both individuals and public health systems in the years to come [41, 47].

3. DENV replication and production in a cell

DENV is a spherical, enveloped virus (**Figure 1**). Mature DENV virions exhibit a smooth surface and measure approximately 50 nm in diameter, whereas immature virions display a spiky surface and are about 60 nm in diameter [48]. In mature DENV, the membrane protein resides beneath the E protein on the virion's surface. Mature DENV possesses a smooth, icosahedral structure. In contrast, immature DENV includes the prM protein, which forms projecting trimers with the E protein, giving it a characteristic "spiky" appearance (**Figure 1**) [49]. DENV comprises a lipid bilayer, an outer shell with well-defined icosahedral symmetry, and a less organized

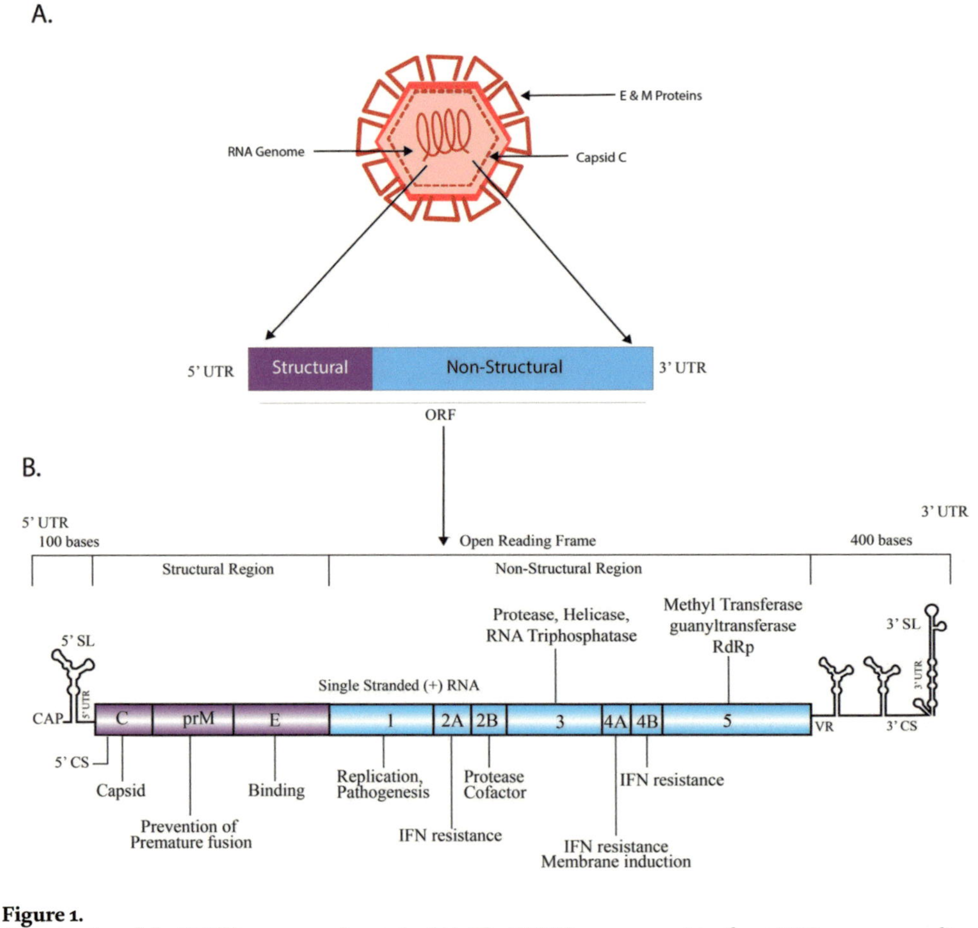

Figure 1.
Organization of the DENV genome and proteins (A). The DENV genome consists of a 5′ UTR, an open reading frame (ORF), and a 3′ UTR. The ORF encodes a polyprotein that is translated into three structural proteins (Capsid (C), Pre-Membrane (PrM), and Envelope (E)) and seven non-structural proteins (NS1, NS2A, NS2B, NS3, NS4A, NS4B, NS5) (B). The 5′UTR contains stem-loop structures in the capsid encoding region. The 3′UTR includes variable sequences, a conserved sequence (CS), and a stem-loop (SL), which are crucial for genome conformational changes and replication. Structural proteins are indicated in purple, and non-structural proteins are indicated in blue.

nucleocapsid containing the capsid proteins [50]. The lipid bilayer and the outer protein shell are situated above the capsid protein. Due to the relatively disorganized nature of the viral RNA compared to the other structural proteins, it can be difficult to distinguish the RNA from the capsid during cryo-electron microscopy imaging [49]. DENV is an enveloped virus with a crucial envelope glycoprotein (E) that mediates receptor binding and fusion, making it a primary target for neutralizing antibodies [50, 51]. DENV's positive-sense, single-stranded RNA genome encodes a polyprotein that is processed into structural proteins, which form the virion, and non-structural proteins, essential for replication. The viral RNA has a 5′ cap but lacks a 3′ poly(A) tail (**Figure 1**) [51]. *Wolbachia's* interactions with DENV proteins are complex and not fully understood, but research has revealed some key mechanisms.

4. Dengue prevention strategies

Dengue prevention centers on minimizing mosquito bites. Personal protection strategies for travelers and residents of endemic areas include the use of insect repellents registered with appropriate regulatory agencies and wearing protective clothing (e.g., long sleeves and pants). Environmental measures such as using screens on windows and doors, air conditioning, and insecticide-treated bed nets can reduce indoor mosquito presence and thus the risk of bites [52]. Critically, source reduction by eliminating mosquito breeding sites—emptying, scrubbing, and covering or removing containers holding standing water around residences—is essential. These mosquito bite prevention measures are recommended for all at-risk individuals, including those who have received a dengue vaccine.

4.1 A new hope for vector control

The potential of *Wolbachia* for insect pest control was recognized decades ago. Early ideas included using *Wolbachia*-induced CI to eliminate *Culex* mosquitoes or to introduce beneficial genes into wild vector populations [21]. Despite this early promise, *Wolbachia* has not yet been widely implemented for vector control. A major obstacle has been the fact that several key vectors of human diseases, including *Ae. aegypti*, the primary dengue vector, are not naturally infected with *Wolbachia*. The *Wolbachia* story took a dramatic turn a decade ago with the development of transinfection techniques. Suddenly, the ability to create stable *Wolbachia* infections in new hosts through delicate embryonic microinjections opened up exciting possibilities. While transinfection is generally more successful between closely related species, and *Wolbachia*'s effects tend to be consistent across different hosts, the real breakthrough came in 2005. Researchers successfully established a stable *Wolbachia* infection in *Ae. aegypti* using a strain from *Ae. albopictus* [53]. This infection not only induced high levels of CI but also spread rapidly through experimental *Ae. aegypti* populations. Soon after, *Ae. aegypti* were successfully double-infected with two different *Wolbachia* strains, again from *Ae. albopictus*, further fueling the growing excitement surrounding this approach [54].

The *Wolbachia* story took another leap forward with the discovery of its direct impact on pathogen transmission in mosquitoes. Previously, *Wolbachia* was primarily considered a gene drive mechanism. However, the development of cell culture adaptation techniques, allowing for transinfection of strains from more distantly related hosts, coupled with the vast diversity of *Wolbachia* strains and their properties, led to new and exciting possibilities [55]. For example, introducing a life-shortening *Wolbachia* strain from *Drosophila* into *Ae. aegypti* effectively halved the mosquito's lifespan in the lab, suggesting that these mosquitoes might not live long enough to transmit dengue [13]. Even more promisingly, this strain also directly inhibited the ability of various pathogens, including the dengue virus, to infect and replicate within *Ae. aegypti* [56]. Subsequent semi-field and field trials in Australia have demonstrated the successful and persistent establishment of *Wolbachia* in wild *Ae. aegypti* populations [57, 58]. These combined effects create a practical foundation for suppressing dengue transmission through the release of *Wolbachia*-infected mosquitoes.

4.2 Virus sequencing as a window into *Wolbachia's* effects

Building on the previous discussion of *Wolbachia* deployment and the need for vigorous evaluation methods, virus sequence analysis offers a powerful tool to further understand the impact of this intervention. Increasing access to viral genome sequence data allows for new methods to understand dengue epidemiology by analyzing changes in viral genetic diversity over time and space [59, 60]. If several types of dengue strains are present before *Wolbachia* is introduced, less local transmission should result in less variety in the virus's genes (a population bottleneck) and longer travel distances for the virus into the area where *Wolbachia* is used. Analyzing viral phylogenetic trees can easily spot new viral strains entering the area, provided enough genetic change has occurred. Earlier studies indicate that dengue virus evolution in Southeast Asia involves viruses frequently moving into the region and transmission happening in very limited areas [60–62]. Although how much detail we can get from viral phylogenetic trees is uncertain, improvements in deep sequencing make this method more powerful. While some viruses from elsewhere will still show up in areas treated with *Wolbachia*, they likely will not stay and spread locally. This should lessen the strong tendency for dengue viruses to cluster geographically in their family trees.

4.3 Gene drive: A powerful tool for mosquito control

Gene drive systems offer a promising avenue for mosquito control, sharing a similar outcome with the "selfish" biased transmission seen with *Wolbachia*. Like *Wolbachia*, gene drives are also "selfish" in that they can spread through populations by favoring their own inheritance, even if they do not necessarily benefit the individual mosquito carrying them [63, 64]. While the mechanisms differ significantly, both gene drives and *Wolbachia* can achieve population-level changes [65]. This is particularly relevant for mosquito control because the pathogens they transmit often have little negative impact on the mosquitoes themselves. Therefore, genes that make mosquitoes resistant to these pathogens (refractory genes) are unlikely to provide a strong evolutionary advantage [66]. While simply releasing large numbers of mosquitoes with these refractory genes (inundative releases) might be sufficient in some cases, linking these genes to a gene drive system is generally necessary for effective large-scale and long-lasting implementation.

5. Mechanisms of DENV blocking by *Wolbachia*

Wolbachia's ability to block viral transmission in mosquitoes may be compromised by changes in mosquito gene expression. While the exact mechanism remains unclear, two primary hypotheses exist: mosquito immune gene activation and competition for host cell resources [67, 68]. Although immune genes are activated in mosquitoes with introduced *Wolbachia*, they do not appear essential for viral blocking in naturally infected mosquitoes. Several antiviral pathways, including JAK-STAT, ROS, and Toll signaling, along with antimicrobial proteins like Vago and Dnmt2, are activated in infected cells [68]. However, a direct link between these pathways and viral blocking has yet to be established. The exonuclease XRN1, involved in viral RNA degradation, is induced in *Wolbachia*-infected cells [69]. While RNA interference is also activated, its role in viral blocking seems less significant [70].

5.1 Resource competition as a viral blocking mechanism

Besides the idea of immune system stimulation, another possibility focuses on the competition between *Wolbachia* and viruses for resources within the host's cells. Studies have shown a link between the amount of *Wolbachia* present and the suppression of viruses, with some data indicating that viruses are kept out of areas where *Wolbachia* is highly concentrated [22, 71]. This points to potential competition for nutrients, particularly amino acids, and other cellular resources [72]. *Wolbachia*'s influence on lipid metabolism, notably cholesterol [73, 74] (essential for dengue virus replication), is another potential competitive factor [75]. Furthermore, *Wolbachia* might physically prevent viruses from accessing cellular organelles crucial for replication [76]. More research is needed to understand whether immune system changes or competition for cellular resources is the primary mechanism by which *Wolbachia* prevents viral replication. A crucial question for determining the ongoing success of viral suppression is how long the immune system remains activated in *Ae. aegypti* mosquitoes carrying *Wolbachia*.

5.2 Secrets of *Wolbachia's* viral blocking: A gene expression perspective

Analyzing the genes that are expressed differently in mosquitoes infected with *Wolbachia* could shed light on how the infection persists and, importantly, how it prevents viral replication. A study examining all the expressed genes (transcriptome analysis) was conducted on *Ae. aegypti* mosquitoes carrying the *w*Mel strain of *Wolbachia*. These mosquitoes were collected after being released in Cairns, Australia. (2011, 2013–2014, and 2017) revealed significant differences in gene expression [77]. Mosquitoes from the 2017 collection showed a considerably higher number of differentially expressed genes (DEGs) compared to those from the earlier releases. This difference does not appear to be linked to overall *Wolbachia* density. While intrinsic population differences are possible, another explanation is that gene expression has become attenuated as the mosquitoes have evolved in response to the *Wolbachia* infection. Attenuation of *Wolbachia*-mediated effects has been observed in other insect species, though *w*Mel-associated traits generally appear phenotypically stable [78]. If this antiviral activity stems from gene expression rather than structural changes induced by *Wolbachia*, the genes responsible are more likely to be consistently differentially expressed across all mosquito release groups. Intriguingly, the 2017 mosquito group displayed a significantly greater number of both up- and downregulated DEGs compared to earlier releases [77].

DEGs with consistently altered expression across all *Wolbachia* release years fell into three main groups: those related to the immune system, metabolism, and cell growth. One possible way *Wolbachia* protects mosquitoes from viruses is by pre-activating or increasing the activity of genes that fight microbes, a process known as innate immune priming [79]. Focusing on immune-related DEGs, Wimalasiri-Yapa et al. [77] highlighted the upregulation of genes involved in pathogen recognition (CTLGA8, alpha-2-macroglobulin, leucine-rich repeat protein), immune signaling pathways like Toll and IMD (GNBP1, PGRP1, uncharacterized protein LOC5577955), and antimicrobial peptides (defensin-C). These findings support the hypothesis that *Wolbachia* primes the mosquito's innate immune system, leading to enhanced antiviral activity through the upregulation of these crucial immune genes.

6. Decoding *Wolbachia's* viral defense strategy

Wolbachia's influence on host physiology, particularly its impact on secondary infections (especially RNA viruses), is a key area of interest. *Wolbachia's* antiviral mechanisms are complex and likely influenced by the host's cellular environment [67]. To study this interaction, Lindsey et al. [80] used a model system and found significant changes in gene expression and isoform usage in *Wolbachia*-infected flies. Their research highlighted key biological processes affected by the presence of the bacteria. *Wolbachia*, viral infection, and their combination significantly alter how genes are spliced into different isoforms. While *Wolbachia's* influence on splicing was also recently observed in wasps [81], splicing is known to be important in host-microbe interactions [82]. It is not yet known whether *Wolbachia* itself influences splicing or if the changes are a response from the mosquito. Regardless of the cause, these splicing variations likely have important consequences because they alter the resulting proteins and their quantities.

Wolbachia infection causes substantial changes in various biological processes of its host. These affected processes include stress responses, protein tagging for degradation, gene expression (both transcription and translation), RNA regulation, metabolism, and cell division control. The changes to the host's metabolism are especially significant [83]. Given *Wolbachia's* reliance on host nutrients and its limited metabolic machinery, it likely reflects a complex interplay [84]. *Wolbachia's* numerous amino acid transporters suggest it actively acquires specific metabolites, potentially leading the host to either compensate for altered amino acid levels or restrict metabolite availability to limit *Wolbachia's* access. *Wolbachia's* amino acid transporters likely disrupt host amino acid levels [84], impacting not only protein synthesis but also other metabolic pathways, such as purine and pyrimidine nucleotide synthesis. Lindsey et al. [80] investigated how the gene *prat2*, involved in purine synthesis, affects the *Wolbachia*-virus-host interaction. The *prat2* expression influenced viral levels, but this effect depended on *Wolbachia's* presence, highlighting the complexity of the system and suggesting multiple factors contribute to viral blocking. In *Wolbachia*-infected flies, where *prat2* is upregulated, reducing *prat2* increases the viral load, supporting the idea that *Wolbachia* creates an antiviral state. The downstream effects of *prat2* changes and how they differ between *Wolbachia*-infected and uninfected flies are unclear. For instance, *prat2* knockdown might increase purine salvage pathway activity, leading to different by-products and intermediates that could affect cellular processes and viral replication. These downstream effects might explain the observed interaction between *Wolbachia*, *prat2* expression, and viral titer. Given the distinct regulation of metabolic pathways by *Wolbachia* and viruses, other genes likely exhibit *Wolbachia*-dependent effects on viral infection.

The observation that nucleotide metabolism mediates the interaction between *Wolbachia* and viruses is particularly compelling, especially considering that many existing antiviral drugs target these same metabolic pathways. Nucleotide metabolism is a key point of interaction between Wolbachia and viruses, as many antiviral drugs target these metabolic pathways. Ribavirin and similar compounds exert broad-spectrum antiviral effects by inhibiting IMP dehydrogenase, an enzyme involved in purine metabolism [85]. Favipiravir, another antiviral, loses effectiveness when purine levels are high [86]. A recently identified broad-spectrum antiviral interferes with pyrimidine metabolism by inhibiting dihydroorotate dehydrogenase (dhod in Drosophila) [87], which was significantly affected by Wolbachia colonization [80]. An excess of pyrimidines counteracts this antiviral effect, restoring viral replication. Additionally, other antivirals, such as brequinar and leflunomide, also target dihydroorotate dehydrogenase, disrupting pyrimidine metabolism and contributing to their broad-spectrum activity. These findings suggest that Wolbachia alters nucleotide metabolism in ways that overlap with antiviral drug mechanisms, revealing potential interactions between bacterial symbiosis and viral infections. Furthermore, a separate class of antivirals, including brequinar, leflunomide, and related compounds, also targets dihydroorotate dehydrogenase and pyrimidine pools, explaining their broad-spectrum antiviral effects [88]. This convergence of *Wolbachia*-virus interactions and antiviral drug targets on nucleotide metabolism underscores the importance of this pathway in antiviral defense and highlights potential avenues for future therapeutic strategies.

Wolbachia genomics has advanced significantly, now providing insights into the molecular interactions between *Wolbachia* and its hosts. The complete genomes of *Wolbachia* strains infecting both arthropods and nematodes have been sequenced, and specific gene variants have been analyzed across numerous strains. Arthropod-infecting *Wolbachia* genomes range from 1.2 to 1.6 million base pairs (Mb), while nematode-infecting *Wolbachia* genomes are smaller, ranging from 0.9 to 1.1 Mb [84, 89]. Arthropod *Wolbachia*, like other obligate intracellular bacteria, have reduced metabolic capabilities, though they can still synthesize nucleotide triphosphates like ATP [84, 89, 90]. Genomic studies have centered on the *wsp* gene (encoding a variable outer membrane protein), ankyrin-repeat proteins, and WO phage genes. Lacking genetic manipulation tools for *Wolbachia*, researchers use comparative genomics to link natural genetic variations to the reproductive alterations they cause in hosts.

6.1 Direct protein-protein interactions

Some studies suggest that *Wolbachia* proteins might directly interact with DENV proteins. One example is the *Wolbachia* surface protein *wsp*, which has been found to interact with a mosquito protein that is also involved in DENV replication. *Wolbachia's* ability to restrict flavivirus replication and transmission in mosquitoes points to its capacity to manipulate host cellular pathways. While interactions between *Wolbachia* and host proteins are known to contribute to endosymbiosis [91], the role of such interactions in *Wolbachia*'s antiviral activity remains understudied. W*sp* is secreted into the host cytoplasm of mosquito cells. Co-immunoprecipitation identified interactions between wsp and two host proteins (Serine/threonine kinases (STK) and SVM), as well as a *Wolbachia* protein (GroEL). STK and SVM are induced in *Wolbachia*-infected and DENV-infected cells and mosquitoes but are downregulated in DENV-infected, *Wolbachia*-superinfected cells [92]. Knockdown of STK, but not SVM, significantly reduces DENV replication *in vitro* and *in vivo*, suggesting a pro-viral role for STK. This downregulation of STK by *Wolbachia* upon DENV infection may contribute to its anti-dengue activity.

Serine/threonine kinases (STKs) play diverse roles, including involvement in bacterial processes like virulence and cell division [93]. The upregulation of STK transcripts in *Wolbachia*-infected cells, even without viral infection, suggests its importance for *Wolbachia's* lifecycle. Given that flavivirus NS5 proteins are phosphorylated, often on serine residues, and that this phosphorylation can influence viral replication [94–96], the observed interaction between *Wolbachia's* WSP and host STK becomes relevant to *Wolbachia's* antiviral activity. While STKs can be co-opted by viruses [97, 98], the downregulation of STK by *Wolbachia* upon DENV infection, coupled with the observed reduction in DENV replication upon STK knockdown, suggests that *Wolbachia* may be manipulating STK to inhibit DENV replication. Essentially, *Wolbachia* appears to be counteracting the pro-viral potential of STK to enhance its antiviral defense against DENV.

To see how STK affects dengue, researchers boosted STK levels in mosquito cells with and without *Wolbachia* using a special RNA [99]. Boosting STK made dengue grow more in both types of cells, confirming that STK helps dengue. However, the boost had a bigger effect in cells *with Wolbachia*. This is likely because dengue itself already raises STK in cells *without Wolbachia*, so adding more STK does not make as much difference. Since *Wolbachia* normally *reduces* STK, these experiments suggest that *Wolbachia* fights dengue by lowering STK; protein dengue needs to replicate well [92]. *Wolbachia*'s surface protein (*wsp*) interacts with a mosquito protein, STK. STK normally boosts dengue replication. However, *Wolbachia* infection lowers STK levels, especially when dengue is also present. Reducing STK hinders dengue, while increasing STK helps it. Thus, *Wolbachia* likely suppresses STK to fight dengue. The wsp binding to STK might also contribute to this effect.

7. Potential for dengue virulence evolution in response to *Wolbachia*

Because *Wolbachia* can alter both viral and mosquito life cycles, it could theoretically influence the evolution of DENV virulence in both humans and mosquitoes. A key question is whether *Wolbachia* might inadvertently select for more virulent DENV strains. Predicting how DENV virulence might evolve in response to *Wolbachia* is complex and requires further investigation. Predicting how DENV virulence will evolve in response to *Wolbachia* is difficult. Current evolutionary models, which usually assume a trade-off between transmission and virulence (measured as host death rate), are not reliable enough. These models often focus on theoretical equilibrium virulence levels and often ignore the many environmental factors that significantly influence disease severity and virulence evolution [100].

Using *Wolbachia* to shorten mosquito lifespan and thereby curb dengue transmission is a limited, short-term solution. Life-shortening *Wolbachia* strains face challenges establishing themselves due to fitness costs [101]. Introducing one strain can also hinder the later introduction of potentially better strains, so only highly promising strains should be introduced. While some *Wolbachia* strains can block dengue transmission, offering a potential eradication strategy, viral evolution could overcome this block. Evidence suggests dengue can evolve to bypass *Wolbachia*'s interference, potentially within a decade. However, *Wolbachia* is also expected to maintain at least partial blocking long-term, and complete blocking is not impossible. Even partial blocking could significantly reduce dengue incidence due to the large human population at risk and relatively low transmission rates [102].

The next critical step in evaluating *Wolbachia*'s potential for dengue control is assessing its efficacy in reducing human infection through medium-scale deployments. The gold standard for this assessment is a cluster randomized trial, a design particularly well-suited for interventions like *Wolbachia* release where individual targeting is impractical [103]. Directly proceeding with a large-scale cluster randomized trial for *Wolbachia*-based dengue control is currently premature for several reasons. First, the optimal *Wolbachia* strain for a given area needs to be determined through field testing, as different strains have varying effects on dengue blocking and mosquito fitness. Second, while deployments in North Queensland offer a starting point, these conditions differ significantly from the large urban centers of Southeast Asia and Latin America, where such trials would likely occur. Third, *Wolbachia* deployment strategies often require adaptive adjustments based on real-time monitoring of release effectiveness and community engagement (e.g., adjusting mosquito release numbers, trap grids, or release locations). A standard cluster randomized trial would restrict such necessary flexibility. Finally, a traditional two-armed trial designed to detect a 50% reduction in dengue with sufficient power would be very large (over 80 clusters, each with ~100 participants) and costly (estimated at US$5–10 million) [103]. These studies would be conducted in various locations, and their results would be combined in a meta-analysis to assess *Wolbachia*'s impact on disease and infection rates. This approach aims to provide sufficient evidence to justify further development and a future definitive efficacy trial.

8. Conclusion

Wolbachia offers a promising new biological approach to controlling dengue by disrupting its transmission. While long-term effectiveness and viral adaptation need further study, current evidence suggests that *Wolbachia's* mechanisms, including immune priming and resource competition, provide a strong defense against the virus. Continued research focusing on strain optimization, long-term impacts, and rigorous evaluation, alongside advancements in gene drive technology and antiviral drugs, holds significant potential for effective and sustainable dengue control.

Abbreviations

Ae	Aedes
CI	cytoplasmic incompatibility
DEGs	differentially expressed genes
DENV	dengue virus
STKs	serine/threonine kinases
wsp	*Wolbachia*'s surface protein

Author details

Iqra Mushtaq, Ammara Chaudhry and Muhammad Sajjad Sarwar*
Department of Zoology, Faculty of Life Sciences, University of Okara, Okara, Pakistan

*Address all correspondence to: mssravian@gmail.com

References

[1] World Health Organization. Dengue and Severe Dengue. 2024. Available from: https://www.who.int/news-room/fact-sheets/detail/dengue-and-severe-dengue

[2] Wilder-Smith A et al. Preventing dengue epidemics during the COVID-19 pandemic. The American Journal of Tropical Medicine and Hygiene. 2020;**103**(2):570-571

[3] World Health Organization. 2024. Available from: https://www.who.int/news-room/questions-and-answers/item/dengue-vaccines

[4] Morrison AC et al. Defining challenges and proposing solutions for control of the virus vector *Aedes aegypti*. PLoS Medicine. 2008;**5**(3):e68

[5] Achee NL et al. A critical assessment of vector control for dengue prevention. PLoS Neglected Tropical Diseases. 2015;**9**(5):e0003655

[6] Moyes CL et al. Contemporary status of insecticide resistance in the major *Aedes* vectors of arboviruses infecting humans. PLoS Neglected Tropical Diseases. 2017;**11**(7):e0005625

[7] European Centre for Disease Prevention and Control (ECDC). 2025. Available from: https://www.ecdc.europa.eu/en/mosquitoborne-diseases

[8] Ye YH et al. The effect of temperature on *Wolbachia*-mediated dengue virus blocking in *Aedes aegypti*. The American Journal of Tropical Medicine and Hygiene. 2016;**94**(4):812-819

[9] Hertig M, Wolbach SB. Studies on rickettsia-like micro-organisms in insects. The Journal of Medical Research. 1924;**44**(3):329-374

[10] Hilgenboecker K et al. How many species are infected with *Wolbachia*?--A statistical analysis of current data. FEMS Microbiology Letters. 2008;**281**(2):215-220

[11] Stouthamer R, Breeuwer JA, Hurst GD. *Wolbachia* pipientis: Microbial manipulator of arthropod reproduction. Annual Review of Microbiology. 1999;**53**:71-102

[12] Ju JF et al. *Wolbachia* supplement biotin and riboflavin to enhance reproduction in planthoppers. The ISME Journal. 2020;**14**(3):676-687

[13] McMeniman CJ et al. Stable introduction of a life-shortening *Wolbachia* infection into the mosquito *Aedes aegypti*. Science. 2009;**323**(5910):141-144

[14] Brownlie JC et al. Evidence for metabolic provisioning by a common invertebrate endosymbiont, *Wolbachia* pipientis, during periods of nutritional stress. PLoS Pathogens. 2009;**5**(4):e1000368

[15] Kambris Z et al. Immune activation by life-shortening *Wolbachia* and reduced filarial competence in mosquitoes. Science. 2009;**326**(5949):134-136

[16] Pan X et al. The bacterium *Wolbachia* exploits host innate immunity to establish a symbiotic relationship with the dengue vector mosquito *Aedes aegypti*. The ISME Journal. 2018;**12**(1):277-288

[17] Duan XZ et al. Recent infection by *Wolbachia* alters microbial communities in wild Laodelphax striatellus populations. Microbiome. 2020;**8**(1):104

[18] Simhadri RK et al. The gut commensal microbiome of *Drosophila*

melanogaster is modified by the endosymbiont *Wolbachia*. mSphere. 2017;**2**(5):e00287-17

[19] Shropshire JD, Leigh B, Bordenstein SR. Symbiont-mediated cytoplasmic incompatibility: What have we learned in 50 years? eLife. 2020;**9**:e61989

[20] Caragata EP et al. *Wolbachia* as translational science: Controlling mosquito-borne pathogens. Trends in Parasitology. 2021;**37**(12):1050-1067

[21] Laven H. Eradication of *Culex* pipiens fatigans through cytoplasmic incompatibility. Nature. 1967;**216**(5113):383-384

[22] Johnson KN. The impact of *Wolbachia* on virus infection in mosquitoes. Viruses. 2015;**7**(11):5705-5717

[23] Gómez M et al. *Aedes aegypti* and Ae. Albopictus microbiome/virome: New strategies for controlling arboviral transmission? Parasites and Vectors. 2022;**15**(1):287

[24] Lewis J et al. Intrinsic factors driving mosquito vector competence and viral evolution: A review. Frontiers in Cellular and Infection Microbiology. 2023;**13**:1330600

[25] Tabachnick WJ. Nature, nurture and evolution of intra-species variation in mosquito arbovirus transmission competence. International Journal of Environmental Research and Public Health. 2013;**10**(1):249-277

[26] Kittayapong P et al. Distribution and diversity of Wolbachia infections in southeast Asian mosquitoes (Diptera: Culicidae). Journal of Medical Entomology. 2000;**37**(3):340-345

[27] Rasgon JL, Scott TW. An initial survey for *Wolbachia* (Rickettsiales: Rickettsiaceae) infections in selected California mosquitoes (Diptera: Culicidae). Journal of Medical Entomology. 2004;**41**(2):255-257

[28] Ricci I et al. Searching for *Wolbachia* (Rickettsiales: Rickettsiaceae) in mosquitoes (Diptera: Culicidae): Large polymerase chain reaction survey and new identifications. Journal of Medical Entomology. 2002;**39**(4):562-567

[29] O'Connor L et al. Open release of male mosquitoes infected with a *Wolbachia* biopesticide: Field performance and infection containment. PLoS Neglected Tropical Diseases. 2012;**6**(11):e1797

[30] Rasić G et al. Using *Wolbachia*-based release for suppression of *Aedes* mosquitoes: Insights from genetic data and population simulations. Ecological Applications. 2014;**24**(5):1226-1234

[31] Bourtzis K et al. More than one rabbit out of the hat: Radiation, transgenic and symbiont-based approaches for sustainable management of mosquito and tsetse fly populations. Acta Tropica. 2016;**157**:115-130

[32] Dyck VA, Hendrichs J, Robinson AS. Sterile Insect Technique: Principles and Practice in Area-Wide Integrated Pest Management. The Hague: Taylor & Francis; 2021

[33] World Health Organization. WHO: Call for Public Consultation-Development of Target Product Profiles (TPPs) for *Wolbachia* Infected *Aedes aegypti* Population Replacement Intervention. 2022. Available from: https://www.who.int/news-room/articles-detail/call-for-public-consultation-development-target-product-profiles-wolbachia-infected-aedes-aegypti-population-replacement-intervention

[34] Campbell LP et al. Climate change influences on global distributions of dengue and chikungunya virus vectors. Philosophical Transactions of the Royal Society of London. Series B, Biological Sciences. 2015;**370**(1665):20140135

[35] Kraemer MU et al. The global distribution of the arbovirus vectors *Aedes aegypti* and Ae. Albopictus. eLife. 2015;**4**:e08347

[36] Messina JP et al. The current and future global distribution and population at risk of dengue. Nature Microbiology. 2019;**4**(9):1508-1515

[37] Soneja S et al. A review of dengue's historical and future health risk from a changing climate. Current Environmental Health Reports. 2021;**8**(3):245-265

[38] Barrera R, Amador M, MacKay AJ. Population dynamics of *Aedes aegypti* and dengue as influenced by weather and human behavior in San Juan, Puerto Rico. PLoS Neglected Tropical Diseases. 2011;**5**(12):e1378

[39] Eder M et al. Scoping review on vector-borne diseases in urban areas: Transmission dynamics, vectorial capacity and co-infection. Infectious Diseases of Poverty. 2018;**7**(1):90

[40] Gubler DJ. Dengue, urbanization and globalization: The unholy trinity of the 21(st) century. Tropical Medicine and Health. 2011;**39**(Suppl. 4):3-11

[41] Reiter P et al. Texas lifestyle limits transmission of dengue virus. Emerging Infectious Diseases. 2003;**9**(1):86-89

[42] Rivera A et al. Travel-associated and locally acquired dengue cases - United States, 2010-2017. MMWR. Morbidity and Mortality Weekly Report. 2020;**69**(6):149-154

[43] Gubler DJ. Dengue and dengue hemorrhagic fever. Clinical Microbiology Reviews. 1998;**11**(3):480-496

[44] Teixeira Mda G et al. Dynamics of dengue virus circulation: A silent epidemic in a complex urban area. Tropical Medicine and International Health. 2002;**7**(9):757-762

[45] Colón-González FJ et al. Projecting the risk of mosquito-borne diseases in a warmer and more populated world: A multi-model, multi-scenario intercomparison modelling study. Lancet Planet Health. 2021;**5**(7):e404-e414

[46] Giovanetti M et al. Emergence of dengue virus serotype 2 cosmopolitan genotype, Brazil. Emerging Infectious Diseases. 2022;**28**(8):1725-1727

[47] Estallo EL et al. Spatio-temporal dynamics of dengue 2009 outbreak in Córdoba City, Argentina. Acta Tropica. 2014;**136**:129-136

[48] Perera R, Kuhn RJ. Structural proteomics of dengue virus. Current Opinion in Microbiology. 2008;**11**(4):369-377

[49] Zhang W et al. Visualization of membrane protein domains by cryo-electron microscopy of dengue virus. Nature Structural Biology. 2003;**10**(11):907-912

[50] Kuhn RJ et al. Structure of dengue virus: Implications for flavivirus organization, maturation, and fusion. Cell. 2002;**108**(5):717-725

[51] Chambers TJ et al. Flavivirus genome organization, expression,

and replication. Annual Review of Microbiology. 1990;**44**:649-688

[52] CDC. Dengue—Prevent Mosquito Bites. Atlanta, GA: Centers for Disease Control and Prevention, National Center for Emerging and Zoonotic Infectious Diseases (NCEZID), Division of VectorBorne Diseases (DVBD); 2019. Available from: https://www.cdc.gov/dengue/prevention/

[53] Xi Z, Khoo CC, Dobson SL. *Wolbachia* establishment and invasion in an *Aedes aegypti* laboratory population. Science. 2005;**310**(5746):326-328

[54] Ruang-Areerate T, Kittayapong P. *Wolbachia* transinfection in *Aedes aegypti*: A potential gene driver of dengue vectors. Proceedings of the National Academy of Sciences of the United States of America. 2006;**103**(33):12534-12539

[55] McMeniman CJ et al. Host adaptation of a *Wolbachia* strain after long-term serial passage in mosquito cell lines. Applied and Environmental Microbiology. 2008;**74**(22):6963-6969

[56] Moreira LA et al. A *Wolbachia* symbiont in *Aedes aegypti* limits infection with dengue, Chikungunya, and plasmodium. Cell. 2009;**139**(7):1268-1278

[57] Hoffmann AA et al. Successful establishment of *Wolbachia* in *Aedes* populations to suppress dengue transmission. Nature. 2011;**476**(7361):454-457

[58] Walker T et al. The wMel *Wolbachia* strain blocks dengue and invades caged *Aedes aegypti* populations. Nature. 2011;**476**(7361):450-453

[59] Rabaa MA et al. Phylogeography of recently emerged DENV-2 in southern Viet Nam. PLoS Neglected Tropical Diseases. 2010;**4**(7):e766

[60] Raghwani J et al. Endemic dengue associated with the co-circulation of multiple viral lineages and localized density-dependent transmission. PLoS Pathogens. 2011;**7**(6):e1002064

[61] Jarman RG et al. Microevolution of dengue viruses circulating among primary school children in Kamphaeng Phet, Thailand. Journal of Virology. 2008;**82**(11):5494-5500

[62] Rabaa MA et al. Frequent in-migration and highly focal transmission of dengue viruses among children in Kamphaeng Phet, Thailand. PLoS Neglected Tropical Diseases. 2013;**7**(1):e1990

[63] Champer J, Buchman A, Akbari OS. Cheating evolution: Engineering gene drives to manipulate the fate of wild populations. Nature Reviews. Genetics. 2016;**17**(3):146-159

[64] Raban RR, Marshall JM, Akbari OS. Progress towards engineering gene drives for population control. The Journal of Experimental Biology. 2020;**223**(Pt Suppl. 1):jeb208181

[65] Alphey LS et al. Opinion: Standardizing the definition of gene drive. Proceedings of the National Academy of Sciences of the United States of America. 2020;**117**(49):30864-30867

[66] Rasgon JL. Multi-locus assortment (MLA) for transgene dispersal and elimination in mosquito populations. PLoS One. 2009;**4**(6):e5833

[67] Lindsey ARI et al. Conflict in the intracellular lives of endosymbionts and viruses: A mechanistic look at *Wolbachia*-mediated pathogen-blocking. Viruses. 2018;**10**(4):141

[68] Terradas G, McGraw EA. *Wolbachia*-mediated virus blocking in the mosquito vector *Aedes aegypti*. Current Opinion in Insect Science. 2017;**22**:37-44

[69] Thomas S et al. *Wolbachia*-mediated virus blocking in mosquito cells is dependent on XRN1-mediated viral RNA degradation and influenced by viral replication rate. PLoS Pathogens. 2018;**14**(3):e1006879

[70] Terradas G, Joubert DA, McGraw EA. The RNAi pathway plays a small part in *Wolbachia*-mediated blocking of dengue virus in mosquito cells. Scientific Reports. 2017;**7**:43847

[71] Lu P et al. *Wolbachia* induces density-dependent inhibition to dengue virus in mosquito cells. PLoS Negleced Tropical Diseases. 2012;**6**(7):e1754

[72] Caragata EP et al. Competition for amino acids between *Wolbachia* and the mosquito host, *Aedes aegypti*. Microbial Ecology. 2014;**67**(1):205-218

[73] Caragata EP et al. Dietary cholesterol modulates pathogen blocking by *Wolbachia*. PLoS Pathogens. 2013;**9**(6):e1003459

[74] Molloy JC et al. *Wolbachia* modulates lipid metabolism in *Aedes* albopictus mosquito cells. Applied and Environmental Microbiology. 2016;**82**(10):3109-3120

[75] Lee CJ et al. Cholesterol effectively blocks entry of flavivirus. Journal of Virology. 2008;**82**(13):6470-6480

[76] White PM et al. Reliance of *Wolbachia* on high rates of host proteolysis revealed by a genome-wide RNAi screen of *Drosophila* cells. Genetics. 2017;**205**(4):1473-1488

[77] Wimalasiri-Yapa B et al. Differences in gene expression in field populations of *Wolbachia*-infected *Aedes aegypti* mosquitoes with varying release histories in northern Australia. PLoS Neglected Tropical Diseases. 2023;**17**(3):e0011222

[78] Ross PA, Hoffmann AA. Fitness costs of *Wolbachia* shift in locally-adapted *Aedes aegypti* mosquitoes. Environmental Microbiology. 2022;**24**(12):5749-5759. DOI: 10.1111/1462-2920.16235

[79] Rancès E et al. The relative importance of innate immune priming in *Wolbachia*-mediated dengue interference. PLoS Pathogens. 2012;**8**(2):e1002548

[80] Lindsey ARI et al. *Wolbachia* and virus alter the host transcriptome at the interface of nucleotide metabolism pathways. MBio. 2021;**12**(1):e03472-20

[81] Wu X et al. Distinct epigenomic and transcriptomic modifications associated with *Wolbachia*-mediated asexuality. PLoS Pathogens. 2020;**16**(3):e1008397

[82] Chauhan K et al. RNA splicing: A new paradigm in host-pathogen interactions. Journal of Molecular Biology. 2019;**431**(8):1565-1575

[83] Newton ILG, Rice DW. The jekyll and hyde symbiont: Could *Wolbachia* Be a nutritional mutualist? Journal of Bacteriology. 2020;**202**(4):e00589-19

[84] Wu M et al. Phylogenomics of the reproductive parasite *Wolbachia* pipientis wMel: A streamlined genome overrun by mobile genetic elements. PLoS Biology. 2004;**2**(3):E69

[85] Leyssen P et al. The predominant mechanism by which ribavirin exerts its antiviral activity in vitro against flaviviruses and paramyxoviruses is mediated by inhibition of IMP dehydrogenase. Journal of Virology. 2005;**79**(3):1943-1947

[86] Furuta Y et al. In vitro and in vivo activities of anti-influenza virus compound T-705. Antimicrobial Agents and Chemotherapy. 2002;**46**(4):977-981

[87] Hoffmann HH et al. Broad-spectrum antiviral that interferes with de novo pyrimidine biosynthesis. Proceedings of the National Academy of Sciences of the United States of America. 2011;**108**(14):5777-5782

[88] Greene S et al. Inhibition of dihydroorotate dehydrogenase by the immunosuppressive agent leflunomide. Biochemical Pharmacology. 1995;**50**(6):861-867

[89] Foster J et al. The *Wolbachia* genome of Brugia malayi: Endosymbiont evolution within a human pathogenic nematode. PLoS Biology. 2005;**3**(4):e121

[90] Fenn K, Blaxter M. *Wolbachia* genomes: Revealing the biology of parasitism and mutualism. Trends in Parasitology. 2006;**22**(2):60-65

[91] Lindsey ARI. Sensing, signaling, and secretion: A review and analysis of systems for regulating host interaction in *Wolbachia*. Genes (Basel). 2020;**11**(7):813

[92] Hussain M, Qi Z, Asgari S. Interaction of the *Wolbachia* surface protein with a novel pro-viral protein from *Aedes aegypti*. MBio. 2025;**16**(1):e0148624

[93] Pereira SF, Goss L, Dworkin J. Eukaryote-like serine/threonine kinases and phosphatases in bacteria. Microbiology and Molecular Biology Reviews. 2011;**75**(1):192-212

[94] Kapoor M et al. Association between NS3 and NS5 proteins of dengue virus type 2 in the putative RNA replicase is linked to differential phosphorylation of NS5. The Journal of Biological Chemistry. 1995;**270**(32):19100-19106

[95] Kim SJ et al. Protein kinase C-related kinase 2 regulates hepatitis C virus RNA polymerase function by phosphorylation. The Journal of Biological Chemistry. 2004;**279**(48):50031-50041

[96] Neddermann P et al. Reduction of hepatitis C virus NS5A hyperphosphorylation by selective inhibition of cellular kinases activates viral RNA replication in cell culture. Journal of Virology. 2004;**78**(23):13306-13314

[97] Johnston JB et al. Role of the serine-threonine kinase PAK-1 in myxoma virus replication. Journal of Virology. 2003;**77**(10):5877-5888

[98] Kaneko T et al. Production of two phosphoproteins from the NS5A region of the hepatitis C viral genome. Biochemical and Biophysical Research Communications. 1994;**205**(1):320-326

[99] Khorkova O et al. Amplifying gene expression with RNA-targeted therapeutics. Nature Reviews. Drug Discovery. 2023;**22**(7):539-561

[100] Vizoso DB, Ebert D. Phenotypic plasticity of host-parasite interactions in response to the route of infection. Journal of Evolutionary Biology. 2005;**18**(4):911-921

[101] Barton NH, Turelli M. Spatial waves of advance with bistable dynamics: Cytoplasmic and genetic analogues of Allee effects. The American Naturalist. 2011;**178**(3):E48-E75

[102] Hughes H, Britton NF. Modelling the use of *Wolbachia* to control dengue fever transmission. Bulletin of Mathematical Biology. 2013;**75**(5):796-818

[103] Wolbers M et al. Considerations in the design of clinical trials to test novel entomological approaches to dengue control. PLoS Neglected Tropical Diseases. 2012;**6**(11):e1937

Chapter 8

Machine Learning and Artificial Intelligence Predictive Models for Viral Genome and Human Proteome Interactions

Priya Hays

Abstract

Viruses are the known causative agents of pandemics that have led to healthcare crises. Understanding viral entry into the host is through deciphering viral replication and production processes involving sequencing of viral genomes. Characterized as host-proteome interactions, visual studies involve X-ray crystallography, CT scanning and magnetic resonance imaging. The interaction of the viral genome and human proteome may effectively be improved by artificial intelligence tools and machine learning methods in terms of increasing sensitivity, specificity, and accuracy. Most of the existing models are deep learning tools that analyze sequence-sequence datasets that predict these interactions, and some use phenotypes derived from the symptomatology that these viruses cause. The COVID-19 virus has been extensively studied and provides the most data for developing these tools. A huge volume of data are now available to predict viral genome-human proteome interactions involving viral replication and transcription processes, such as the lytic cycle and lysogeny that lead to host cell infectivity. Understanding of these processes would lead to predicting genomic-proteomic patterns that would greatly improve accuracy.

Keywords: viral replication cycle, artificial intelligence, convolutional neural networks, COVID-19, Mpox, hepatitis

1. Introduction

Single-strand positive sense RNA viruses like COVID-19, are recent causes of global pandemics leading to public health crises, resulting in mortality on a large scale, which may be exacerbated by climate change [1]. Viruses have been characterized as non-living due to their dependence on cellular hosts for viral replication and reproduction. The pandemic as a result of COVID-19, due to its ssRNA genome, and its complex pathogen entry and regulatory processes relying on pathogen-pathogen interactions, has led to formulations conferring the possible classification as a living entity [2].

This is augmented by artificial intelligence strategies that led to an understanding of the evolutionary advantages of this virus. Classical machine learning (ML) modeling involves unsupervised and supervised training of datasets to model patterns in data and also involves deep learning, a subset of ML for pattern learning with enormous accuracy [3]. The data and information generated may be crucial for prevention of pandemics.

The impetus for the use of artificial intelligence (AI), machine learning (ML), deep learning (DL), and computational methods for characterizing viral and host interaction became all the more urgent with the emergence of the COVID-19 and the pandemic, which led to new understandings for investigating the nature of virus-host cell interaction. Research has generated massive genetic and molecular datasets in predicting viral and host interactions using AI and ML [4].

Experimental methods such as X-ray crystallography or other imaging modalities such as magnetic resonance imaging and CT scans are tools to determine the viral-host atomic properties through visual representation; however, this has seen limitations such as achieving high resolution and subjective interpretation, prone to diagnostic error in interpretation, with experimental validation of host-pathogen interactions (HPI) being also limited by cost*. Expertise and clinical experience may not always be available. Artificial intelligence tools can overcome these limitations through "rich structural datasets" through proteomic analysis.* Computation modeling becomes useful through predicting HPI through the human proteome. **Figure 1** shows the workflow for taking raw data, performing training and validation on the data, and outputting trained models. This workflow serves as the paradigm for predicting viral infectivity through the use of machine learning models outlined in this book chapter.

AI and ML tools can process huge volumes of data, detect patterns in the data and learn from them through training and validation, and provide predictive models that can predict infection and control the pandemic spread of the virus.* By simulating human intelligence processes through machines and algorithmic methods that learn and improve from data, machine learning models can be constructed. Deep Learning, or DL, employs neural networks such as convolutional neural networks and artificial neural networks that analyze data parameters [5]. An example of ML, data analysis,

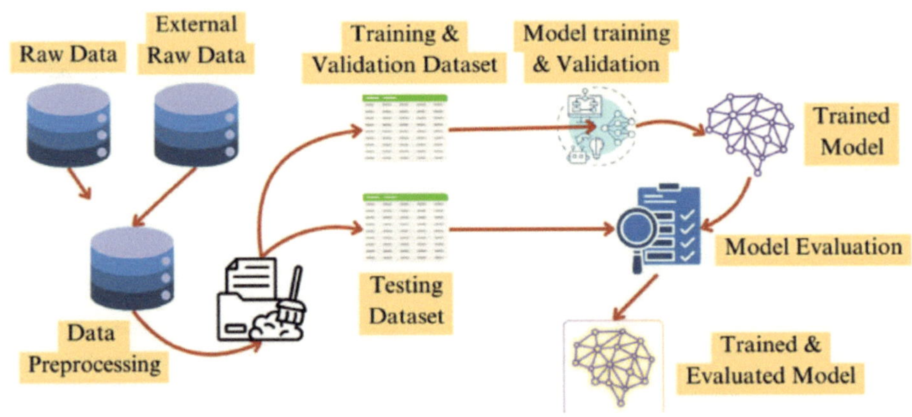

Figure 1.
Shows the workflow for taking raw data, performing training and validation on the data, and outputting trained models (adapted from Gawande et al.) (Permission to reuse under Creative Commons CC BY 4.0).

and advanced AI models when applied to clinical virology (that investigates the genetics of viral proteins) is to construct disease transmission models, determine impacts of pandemic outbreaks, and forecast them accurately. Applications include epidemic detection and patient tracking [6].

AI and ML are already reported to perform as well or better than humans in disease diagnostics and "outperforming radiologists in identifying malignant tumors as well as aiding researchers in the formulation of cohorts in costly clinical trials." As Kaur et al. state, "As one of the most common forms of artificial intelligence, machine learning is a statistical approach for fitting and training models with data" [7].

As one account states:

> *"Machine learning, a subset of AI, facilitates algorithms in learning from data without explicit programming. Instead of relying solely on hard-coded rules, machine learning algorithms construct predictive models by identifying patterns within extensive datasets. As more data are incorporated, these models continuously update to enhance their performance in specified tasks such as classification, regression, and clustering. Commonly used machine learning algorithms include linear regression, logistic regression, naive Bayes classifiers, the k-nearest neighbors algorithm, support vector machines, decision trees (DTs), and neural networks, each with its own strengths, weaknesses, and ap- plication scenarios. Selection of the most suitable machine learning technique is crucial to harnessing the potential of AI in various fields. As research advances, new and hybrid algorithms are being actively developed and applied to address real-world problems" [8].*

This book chapter will review the literature in this field and describe new insights and models into predicting the mechanism of pathogenic viruses such as SARS-CoV-2 and elaborate on artificial intelligence and machine learning models for the monkeypox virus, or Mpox, and Hepatitis infection. According to one analysis, the models must reflect the complex replicative processes of viruses and the transcriptional and translational machinery for host cell appropriation. The computational models must also encompass the entire host cell-viral interactome [9]. One study sought to understand the protein-protein interactions of host viral infectivity by leveraging heterogeneous HPC resources to develop a generalizable AI-driven workflow that explored molecular systems that were time-dependent [2].

A PubMed search was conducted using the following search terms "COVID-19" and "Machine Learning" and "Artificial Intelligence" and "Predictive Models" and "Hepatitis B" and "Machine Learning" and "Artificial Intelligence" and "Predictive Modeling" and "Pandemic Control" and "Clinical Virology."

2. Predictive models and viral genomic-human proteomic interactions

The ACE2 receptor serves as the host receptor for COVID-19 entry by binding its spike protein into human cells that leads to either viral lysogenic activity for long-term integration into the host genome or viral lysis involving the overtaking of host cellular activities and functions. A large inflammatory systemic reaction results in respiratory system dysfunction and physical symptoms associated with infection, such as pneumonia, fever, cough, and dyspnea.

This process is subject to predictive modeling by machine learning methods and deep learning, part of artificial intelligence tools. ANN, or artificial neural networks, and CNN, convolutional neural networks, are computational modeling methods that are able to predict host-pathogen interactome and may result in prevention of the spread of viruses [2].

RNA structure is conserved across the virus's genome, and with the aid of a deep learning tool, repurposed drugs were effective against the virus's replication and production by predicting host proteins that would serve as targets for these medications [10, 11].

A machine learning tool termed VHIP Viral Host Interaction Predictor could predict "host-pathogen interactions" through a trained dataset inputted from host and viral genomes, resulting in a Viral Host Range network, which has an 87.8% accuracy prediction rate, providing for holistic comparison of host prediction tools [12].

One study also reported on the validity of machine learning to predict host pathogenicity entry through immune escape data and also showed that AI's ability to study the viral spike glycoprotein leads to production of the early vaccines. Multiple algorithms that involved Random Forest and logistic regression showed that ML can predict cell entry of the Ebola virus using the ML-based EBOLApred [3].

Independent datasets, including positive and negative datasets, were produced in one computational modeling study to predict SARS-CoV-2 human protein interactions. SVM, or Support Vector Machine, is the supervised machine learning algorithm that trains the datasets. Accuracy was 72.33%, while specificity and precision were 74.41 and 72.41%, respectively, when compared to all other computational models, and with one database, prediction analysis improved to 3603 host protein interactions. Casalino et al. developed an AI workflow generalizable to investigate the mechanisms of infectivity of the virus's spike glycoprotein or an AI-driven multi-simulation framework to determine spike dynamics [2].

3. Specific models for determining and predicting infectivity

3.1 COVID-19

Yakimovich reported on a viral case for machine learning and artificial intelligence understanding for host-pathogen interactions and conducted a review on large language models developed for analyzing such interactions including ML for natural language processing (NLP). A COVID-19 research dataset was developed called CORD-19, which was used for understanding protein pairs and genes of the coronavirus [1].

DeepHPI is a computational platform that posits to accurately predict host-pathogen interactions through visualization of protein-protein interactions of human viruses. Convolutional neural networks were used for HPI prediction to lead to better prediction of pandemics while circumventing the labor-intensive methods for investigating HPIs. The DeepHPI is the first tool for utilizing convolutional neural networks for predicting HPIs and thereby potentially preventing pandemics. This model was unique in that it used a quantitative analysis for correlating viral processes with its entry into the cellular host and protein-protein interactions and is also significant since multiple user requests can be accommodated on a web server. Positive datasets were generated on PPIs, augmented by mass spectrometry. Negative datasets termed Neglog, InterSPPI, and NegaTome were also generated to decrease false positives. CNNs were also used for feature extraction and to extract refined patterns. Sensitivity and accuracy were 0.9351/0.9398 and 0.9929/0.9931. Modeling of HPIs was also conducted. "For the human–virus dataset, MCC values ranged from 0.6539 (InterSPPI) to 0.9607 (Negatome) in cross-validation and from 0.6715 (InterSPPI) to 0.9671 (Negatome) in independent testing" [13].

DeepViral is a neural network model that predicts host-pathogen interactions through protein-protein sequences and through the disease phenotype itself (i.e., signs and symptoms), serving as an improvement over predicting through sequence-based methods. The neural network model uses supervised methods to predict HPI through sequence analysis and phenotypic characteristics of the virus.

The molecular mechanisms underlying the infectious disease pathogenesis could be better understood, leading to novel drug discovery and drug repurposing as well. Experimental validation of these protein hubs and interactions proves time-consuming and predicting HPI, paving the way for computational prediction of candidate interactions with the human proteome as a complementary approach. In this approach, phenotypes were created by PathoPhenoDB, "a database of manually curated and text-mined associations of pathogens, infectious diseases and phenotypes," and SARS-CoV-2 interactions were detected through 332 PHIs from 27 viral proteins, and to represent the human proteome, phenotypes were generated from the Human Phenotype Ontology database and their associated functions from the Gene Ontology database. The significance of this model was in its joint prediction of HPIs through sequences and phenotypes due to immune-mediated responses that were trained on protein sequences and found that inclusion of the phenotypes predicted the interaction of the viral genomic sequences with protein sequences, since in a clinical context, protein functions are depleted. The authors also reported on several studies the utilized phenotypes and sequence interactions of HPIs to predict signs and symptoms [14].

3.2 Mpox virus

Mpox is an orthopoxvirus that causes a smallpox-like illness, primarily in Central and Western Africa. Transmitted through both the circulatory and respiratory system, most cases are resolved through symptomatic management, with a fatality rate of 3–5%. Antiviral treatments are administered for severe infections. The Mpox genome is being carefully studied to reveal genomic characteristics for understanding its viral replication and production. Its genome is a linear double-stranded DNA genome composed of hairpin loops and inverted tandem repeats, and its transcription factors are protected by an outer membrane. Viral replication takes in the cytoplasm of the host cell through cell-associated virions. Diagnosis is made through routine RT-PCR of its DNA polymerase gene (E9L) and through restriction fragment length polymorphism analysis and whole genome sequencing and next-generation sequencing [12]. One report also revealed how AI and ML led to the diagnosis of Mpox (**Figure 2**) [16].

Artificial intelligence tools have been harnessed to improve accuracy in the diagnosis of radiological graphs and pathological specimens and have proven relevant in cancer by decreasing intra-observer and interobserver variability. The algorithms and statistical models lead to an understanding of the patterns of enriched datasets that enable predictions that aid in decision-making. An artificial intelligence tool for accurate prediction of Mpox genomic proteomic interaction would involve supervised training of datasets through a convolutional neural network leading to sensitivity and specificity values and accuracy rates for predicting infection and infectivity rates. Genomic-proteomic interactions could be further identified, analyzed, and predicted [17].

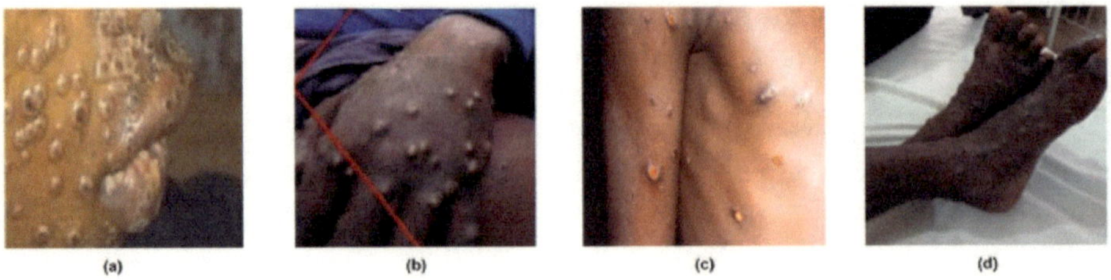

Figure 2.
Pictures of Mpox virus infection in patients (adapted from Chadaga et al.) [15]. Permission to reuse under Creative Commons CC BY 4.0.

Chadaga et al. performed a systematic review of artificial intelligence techniques of the Mpox virus, which can be used to detect clinical disease patterns and life-threatening information through data analysis, in effect to classify skin lesions. They report on "[a]pplying transfer learning to "Monkeypox2022" [that] used a pretrained modified VGG-16, a type of convolutional neural network (CNN), to classify mpox from other classes, attaining accuracy rates ranging from 78 to 97%." A CNN-based model was also developed to classify skin lesions into eight disease classes compared with a pretrained model with accuracy and average precision of 87 and 85%, respectively, and DL was also used to classify Mpox skin lesions. Ahsen et al. studied six DL models to acquire an accuracy of 95 and 97% for discerning Mpox lesions. Saleh et al. used data mining and ML techniques to also classify Mpox lesions [15]. **Table 1** provides the results of the systematic review.

An artificial intelligence model for diagnosing skin lesions would lead to the prediction of the Mpox viral host interactions by training sequence datasets. Such a model would entail developing databases for Mpox genes and protein sequences as well as gene ontologies and utilizing these databases for understanding phenotypic characteristics. HPIs may be predicted through the DL model that provides a neural network architecture that would generate patterns for these interactions, leading to the prevention of potential disease outbreaks.

3.3 Acute and chronic hepatitis infection

Kim et al. used machine learning models to predict hepatitis B or C virus infection in diabetic patients and declared that "machine learning has emerged as a promising alternative to traditional hepatitis screening strategies in recent years." Due to imbalance between hepatitis and non-hepatitis patients, SMOTE, or a synthetic minority oversampling technique, was applied to the dataset prior to establishing a machine

Classifier	Accuracy	AUC	Precision	Recall	F1-score
RF	**0.9944**	**0.9986**	**0.9946**	**0.9954**	**0.9944**
SVM	0.8546	0.9241	0.9821	0.7248	0.7684
AdaBoost	0.903	0.9514	0.9759	0.8319	0.8515

Bold represents the best performing indicator.

Table 1.
(Adapted from Fan et al.) [18] Permission to reuse under Creative Commons CC BY 4.0.

learning method. In order to train and test the model following data normalization, machine learning models were applied [19].

Data collected from the NHANES database was analyzed by machine learning algorithms for detecting hepatitis B and C in diabetic patients in their latent state without serological values. Least absolute shrinkage and selection operator (LASSO), support vector machine (SVM), Random Forest (RF), and eXtreme Gradient Boosting (XGBoost), along with stacked ensemble model, provided quantitative values for sensitivity and specificity to predict infection. Among the best performance prediction models, according to the analysis, LASSO showed the highest predictive performance (AUC-ROC = 0.810) rather than other models, and socioeconomic factors such as illicit drug use, poverty, and race were high-ranking predictor factors for developing hepatitis. The sensitivity of all four models was low; however, the specificity of LASSO at 0.993 was the highest. LASSO also outperformed the other models in terms of precision and other evaluation metrics. Predictive performance was improved by a "stacking ensembles algorithm" in which the accuracy was 0.945, specificity was 0.958, and sensitivity was 0.500. Hyperparameter optimization was also performed to enhance the performance of the machine learning algorithms and "involves selecting the most suitable parameter values from a given parameter space, allowing for the optimization of model complexity" by identifying parameters that cannot be learned from the algorithm themselves (**Table 2**) [19].

Fan et al. developed a machine learning model to predict hepatitis in patients based on serological data that improved upon existing black box machine learning models, including Random Forest, Support Vector Machine (SVM), and AdaBoost. They found that the learning models had varying effects on predicting infection, with SVM having the worst prediction results leading to early misdiagnosis of hepatitis C patients as blood donors, leading investigators not to recommend implementing it in clinical practice for early diagnosis. AdaBoost also has poor predictive power as being the most likely to diagnose blood donors as hepatitis C patients, leading to unnecessary panic. On the other hand, RF was found to be the best-performing model among them.

Algorithm	Sensitivity	Specificity	Precision	F1 score	Accuracy
Without hyperparameter tuning					
RF	0.683	0.903	0.857	0.802	0.760
SVM	0.791	0.916	0.889	0.837	0.859
XGBoost	0.705	0.882	0.836	0.800	0.765
LASSO	0.591	0.898	0.831	0.756	0.691
With hyperparameter tuning					
RF	0.461	0.978	0.400	0.429	0.962
SVM	0.500	0.990	0.600	0.545	0.976
XGBoost	0.500	0.968	0.316	0.387	0.954
LASSO	0.500	0.993	0.667	0.571	0.978

(Adapted from Kim et al.) [19] Permission to reuse under Creative Commons CC BY 4.0.

Table 2.
Sensitivity, specificity and accuracy values resulting from algorithms to detect Hepatitis infection in diabetic patients without and with hyperparameter testing.

Classifier	Accuracy	AUC	Precision	Recall	F1-score
RF	**0.9148**	**0.9895**	0.9008	**0.9277**	**0.9052**
SVM	0.7298	0.7662	**0.9504**	0.5207	0.5545
AdaBoost	0.771	0.8236	0.9136	0.6481	0.6571

Bold represents the best performing indicator.
The authors chose the Bayesian optimized RF as the classifier for hepatitis diagnosis (adapted from Fan et al.) [18]

Table 3.
Tables 2 *and* **3** *show the performance comparison of the three classifiers in the UCI dataset. Random Forest (RF) has an accuracy of 0.9944 and an AUC value of 0.9986, being performing the best among all five evaluation indicators, which is recapitulated in the independent testing set when comparing the performance of three classifiers, whereby overall RF still performs the best.*

The authors adopted a Bayesian-optimized RF as the classification algorithm. One of them outlined here is the Local Interpretable Model-Agnostic Explanations with stability "(LIME_stabilitly)" to provide local explanations for the model. The authors describe the model LIME as "a black-box model interpretation method," interpreting the model by providing one that behaves similar to the original model. They describe their model as approximating the black box model "by using a simple function g around a point x, where g must belong to the class of interpretable models G. Each model corresponds to a specific input point x, only around x are the predictions of the interpretable model guaranteed to be very close to the black box model. This property determines the ability of LIME to act as a local interpretable tool," surpassing the black box model in interpretation (**Table 3**).

As Fan et al. state, "[t]he interpretability makes the prediction process of the model transparent, allowing medical workers without specialized knowledge to understand the prediction process of the prediction model, and helps accelerate the process of machine learning-based hepatitis prediction models to clinical use" (**Figure 3**) [18].

Liver fibrosis as a result of chronic hepatitis B infection was further made amenable to machine learning models that used a decision tree method to analyze serum markers

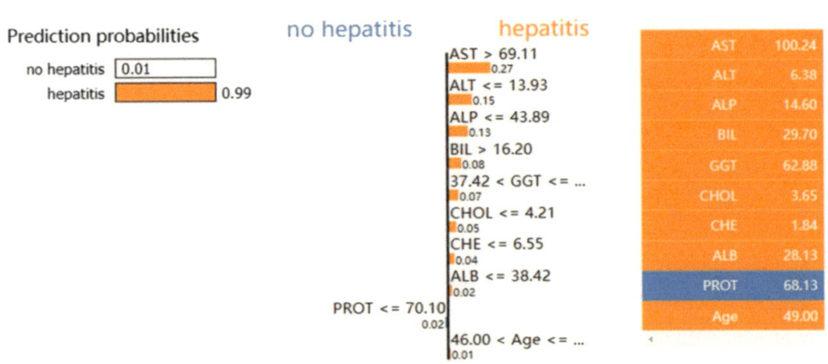

Figure 3.
Indicates that, with AST, ALT, ALP, and BIL being measures of liver function through quantification of liver enzymes and the most critical discriminatory factors, the model has 99% confidence that leads to the conclusion that the patient is a hepatitis patient. Their data also explain the clinical reference basis for the ability to judge and discriminate between positive and negative cases of hepatis provided by the model (adapted from Fan et al.) [18]. Permission to reuse under Creative Commons CC BY 4.0.

Cohorts	ML Model	APRI	FIB-4
Cirrhosis(F4) AUC			
Training cohort	0.944	0.67	0.717
Validation cohort	0.933	0.69	0.735
Advanced fibrosis(F3) AUC			
Training cohort	0.907	0.604	0.567
Validation cohort	0.931	0.63	0.695
Significance fibrosis(F2) AUC			
Training cohort	0.891	0.515	0.527
Validation cohort	0.876	0.559	0.551
Early stage of fibrosis(F0.1) AUC			
Training cohort	0.898	0.602	0.615
Validation cohort	0.906	0.651	0.681

(Adapted from Zhang et al.) [20]. Permission to reuse under Creative Commons CC BY 4.0.

Table 4.
Comparison of the performance of the ML model versus traditional statistical models APRI and FIB-4 in terms of accuracy rates in both training and validation cohorts in stages F1-F4 of chronic hepatic fibrosis.

for indications of liver fibrosis. Results included the prediction of liver fibrosis stages in both the training cohort (AUC 0.898 (F0–1), (0.891 (F2), 0.907 (F3), 0.944 (F4)) and validation cohort (AUC 0.906 (F0–1), 0.876 (F2), 0.931 (F3), 0.933 (F4)). Serological biomarkers on which the constructed DNA model was based were HBV-DNA, platelet, "thrombin time, international normalized ratio," and albumin to assess liver fibrosis.

As the authors concluded that they designed a predictive model based on machine learning in the multicenter study in order to provide accurate assessments of liver fibrosis stage of chronic hepatitis B patients when compared with traditional statistical models such as FIB-4 or APRI, the ML model they developed was easy to process and also demonstrated significant improvements in the field in the evaluation of liver fibrosis as a result of chronic hepatitis B infection. The authors also compared their results to the reference standard of liver biopsy and posit that the ML model they developed provided similar results leading to diagnostic efficacy, being simple, easy-to-use, and an accurate tool for the evaluation of liver fibrosis (**Table 4**) [20].

4. Discussion

Viruses are the known causative agents of recent pandemic outbreaks and have resulted in catastrophic mortality and worldwide crises, with COVID-19 being the most studied example. Understanding viral host interaction processes is a focus of these efforts. Experimental methods such as X-ray crystallography that lead to visual characterizations have been used to identify these processes. AI and ML tools are now being used to circumvent some of the limitations of these methods and develop models of these processes. Patterns generated through generated datasets of sequences as well as infectious disease phenotypes as shown by the DeepViral model and DeepHPI models can predict viral infectivity patterns and lead to the prevention of these outbreaks.

As early as 2020, artificial intelligence and machine learning tools such as SVM were shown to be a robust classifier of use in the COVID-19 pandemic with 100% sensitivity and specificity values in predicting infection [7]. Gawande et al. present an account of how AI-enabled dynamic models were built through ML and DL techniques to monitor the pandemic through screening, forecasting contact tracing and, enhancing diagnostic development. They specifically cite.

"notable models such as the Multi-Task Deep Model, Cog-Mol (Controlled Generation of Molecules), COVID-Net, Random Forest Model(RF), Time-Dependent Susceptible-Infected-Recovered(SIR), DarkCOVIDNet, Support Vector Regression(SVR), and Stacking-Ensemble Models," with the caveat that acquiring more varied datasets is needed to confirm how applicable these AI-based approaches are, such as ResNet-101, which achieved a 99.51% accuracy in distinguishing COVID-19 infection [21].

In the need for the prediction of disease progression and disease outcomes, a number of ML models have emerged in which DL systems on CT images and clinical data have been used. COVID-19 patients who underwent imaging and CT image segmentation techniques were used to identify lung lesions. These authors used DL to predict progression to adverse outcomes including ICU admission and the need for mechanical ventilation. Decision trees have also been constructed based on clinical indicators such as C-reactive protein and lactate dehydrogenase to predict mortality in high-risk patients and prioritize them [8].

Predictive modeling is also being developed for understanding how the virus spreads and enabling health systems to prepare for peak transcription and limitation of outbreaks. One account states that the faster the prediction takes place, the faster protective measures and targeted measures can take place, corresponding to a critical response. Accurate prediction can enable isolation and quarantine procedures for pending treatment.

According to Różyło-Kalinowska and Orhan, predictive ML models include "adaptive neuro-fuzzy interference system (ANFIS), autoregressive integrated moving average (ARIMA), multilayer perception (MLP), long short-term memory (LSTM), the latter in combination with natural language processing (NLP)" exceed in performance traditional statistical modeling with good short-term forecasting, with further studies needed to validate long-term efficacy [22].

Acknowledgements

P.H. wishes to thank the Editors at IntechOpen for their assistance with this manuscript.

Conflict of interest

There is nothing to declare.

P.H. designed and wrote the manuscript in its entirety.

Future directions

AI and ML modeling of viral processes, which were driven by the COVID-19 pandemic, is now a prolific field, with data scientists and bioinformaticians deeply involved in predicting various aspects of the specific viruses described here, including COVID-19, Mpox, and hepatitis. Future research may be directed to bioinformaticians and data scientists to use AI, ML, and DL tools to enhance the accuracy of these models for better prediction.

Author details

Priya Hays
Geisel School of Medicine, Dartmouth College, Hanover, NH, United States

*Address all correspondence to: priya.hays@outlook.com

References

[1] Yakomovich A. Machine learning and artificial intelligence for the prediction of host–pathogen interactions: A viral case. Infection and Drug Resistance. 2021;**14**:3319-3326

[2] Casalino L, Dommer A, Gaieb Z, Barros EP, Sztain T, et al. AI-driven multiscale simulations illuminate mechanisms of SARS-CoV-2 spike dynamics. Supercomputing. 2020:20, Virtual

[3] Stefano G, Kream R. Artificial intelligence in biological sciences. Life 2022. Viruses broaden the definition of life by genomic incorporation of artificial intelligence and machine learning. Processes. Current Neuropharmacology. 2022;**20**:1888-1893

[4] Bhardwaj D, Bhardwaj A, Kishore S, Pandey DK. Artificial intelligence in biological sciences. Life. 2022;**12**:1430

[5] Padhi A, Agarwal A, Saxena SK, Katoch CDS. Transforming clinical virology with AI, machine learning and deep learning: A comprehensive review and outlook. VirusDisease. 2023;**34**(3):345-355

[6] Misra NK, Das S, Satpathy S, Addula SR, Trivedi MC. COVID-19 pandemic: A worldwide critical review with the machine learning model-based prediction. Journal of The Institution of Engineers (India): Series B. 2025;**106**(1):339-349

[7] Kaur I, Behl B, Aleya L, Rahman H, Kumar A, et al. Artificial intelligence as a fundamental tool in management of infectious diseases and its current implementation in COVID-19 pandemic. Environmental Science and Pollution Research. 2021;**28**:40515-40532

[8] Lv C, Guo W, Yin X, Liu L, Huang X, et al. Innovative applications of artificial intelligence during the COVID-19 pandemic. Infectious Medicine. 2024;**3**:100095

[9] Elste J, Saini A, Mejia-Alvarez R, Mejía A, Millán-Pacheco C, et al. Significance of artificial intelligence in the study of virus–host cell interactions. Biomolecules. 2024;**14**:911

[10] Sun et al. In vivo structural characterization of the SARS-CoV-2 RNA genome identifies host proteins vulnerable to repurposed drugs. Cell. 2021;**184**:1865-1883

[11] Karabulut OC, Karpuzcu BA, Türk E, Ibrahim AH, Süzek BE. MLAdVInfect: A machine-learning based adenoviral infection predictor. Frontiers in Molecular Biosciences. 2021;**8**:647424

[12] Bastien GE, Cable RN, Batterbee C, Wing AJ, Zaman L, Duhaime MB. Virus-host interactions predictor (VHIP): Machine learning approach to resolve microbial virus-host interaction networks. PLoS Computational Biology. 2024;**20**(9):1-21

[13] Kaundal R, Loaiza CD, Duhan N, Flandeep N. HPI: A comprehensive deep learning platform for accurate prediction and visualization of host–pathogen protein–protein interactions. Briefings in Bioinformatics. 2022;**23**(3):1-11

[14] Liu-Wei W, Kafkas CJ, Dimonaco NJ, Tegne J, Hoehndor R. DeepViral: Prediction of novel virus–host interactions from protein sequences and infectious disease phenotypes. Bioinformatics. 2021;**37**(17):2722-2729

[15] Chadaga K, Prabhu S, Sampathila N, Nireshwalya S, Katta SS, et al. Application of artificial intelligence techniques for monkeypox: A systematic review. Diagnostics. 2023;**13**:824

[16] Alakunle E, Moens U, Nchinda G, Okeke MI. Monkeypox virus in Nigeria: Infection biology, epidemiology, and evolution. Viruses. 2020;**12**:1257

[17] Hays P. Artificial intelligence in cytopathological applications for cancer: A review of accuracy and analytic validity. European Journal of Medical Research. 2024;**29**:553

[18] Fan Y, Lu X, Sun G. IHCP: Interpretable hepatitis C prediction system based on black-box machine learning models. BMC Bioinformatics. 2023;**24**:333

[19] Kim S-H, Park SH, Lee H. Machine learning for predicting hepatitis B or C virus infection in diabetic patients. Scientific Reports. 2023;**13**:21518

[20] Zhang C, Shu Z, Chen S, Peng JJ, Zhao Y, et al. A machine learning-based model analysis for serum markers of liver fibrosis in chronic hepatitis B patients. Scientific Reports. 2024;**14**:12081

[21] Gawande MS, Zade N, Kumar P, Gundewar S, Weerarathna IN, Verma P. The role of artificial intelligence in pandemic responses: From epidemiological modeling to vaccine development. Molecular Biomedicine. 2025;**6**:1

[22] Różyło-Kalinowska I, Orhan K. Applications of machine learning and artificial intelligence in the COVID-19 pandemic. In: Orhan K, Jagtap R, editors. Artificial Intelligence in Dentistry. Cham, Switzerland: Springer Nature Publishing. pp. 247-257